The Hypothalamus Handbook

*Your Tool to Discovering the Root of Your Health
Issues and Finally Healing Your Body,
Mind, and Soul*

Deborah Maragopoulos FNP

D1719816

Genesis Health Products, Inc Ojai, California

Get your Hypothalamus Handbook gifts here: GenesisGold.com/HH

For my granddaughter Benji:

May we continue to improve health care for your generation

Acknowledgements

In writing a book of this depth, there are so many people that play a part. I want to express my deepest gratitude for all of my patients spanning over three decades. You have helped me formulate my focus on healing the hypothalamus and inspired me to design therapies for hypothalamic dysfunction. Thank you for your faith in me, for your feedback, and for your love.

Thank you also to my team. Without you, I never could have written this book while also consulting with patients and running multiple businesses!

To my right-hand girl, Gabriela Tapia - my beloved assistant and expert Customer Service Rep: Thank you for allowing me to focus on sharing my wisdom.

To my Operations Manager, Amber Kinney, and her team at The AK Collective: Thank you for helping me organize this content and get it to publication. Your ongoing support amplifies my efforts to provide education on the hypothalamus - which offers life-changing results to multitudes of people who need help. Thank you for getting us here!

To my children, Jarys and Kyra: You have always been my inspiration to look for the deeper roots of health issues and model healing lifestyle choices.

Finally, the deepest gratitude to my beloved husband of 40 years: Steve, without your loving support, I never would have been able to finish this project. Thank you for always being there, for supporting my every endeavor, and for helping make my dreams come true.

Contents

Part Three
How to Heal Your Hypothalamus

Part Four
For Healthcare Providers

Introduction

Why write a hypothalamus handbook? What the heck is the hypothalamus anyway? Why try to educate the public and healthcare providers about the importance of paying attention to the hypothalamus and healing it?

Because after over 30 years of helping the hormonally challenged get back in balance, I have found that the majority of the time the root of the issue is hypothalamus dysfunction. Very rarely are the lower endocrine glands at fault for the myriad of symptoms my patients suffer.

It's not so simple an answer just to prescribe someone with low energy and hypothyroidism thyroid replacement therapy for the rest of their life without getting to the root issue of a potential hypothalamic-pituitary-thyroid axis miscommunication.

It's inadequate to treat chronic fatigue patients with mitochondrial support alone without addressing their hypothalamic dysfunction because the hypothalamus controls metabolism at the cellular level.

It's not enough to treat adrenal fatigue with glandulars and adaptogens if you do not address their hypothalamic-pituitary-adrenal axis and nourish their hypothalamus with what's necessary to create the master hormone to stimulate normal circadian adrenal function and a healthy stress response.

It's a shame to over prescribe sedatives and sleep aids and not address the root issue of hypothalamic dysfunction in sleep disorders since the hypothalamus controls circadian rhythm and sleep.

There is not a one size fits all prescription. But there is a way to nourish your hypothalamus so that it can get itself back into balance and communicate with your entire endocrine system, your neurological system, and your immune system so you can finally achieve optimal health.

Your hypothalamus' job is to help you survive. Unfortunately, if it doesn't get the nutrients it needs, if your body cannot detoxify toxins appropriately, if you don't get the sleep that you need, if you don't follow a healthy circadian lifestyle, if you're not active, if your mindset is not healing, it is difficult to balance your hypothalamus.

I decided to address hypothalamus concerns when in spite of my best intentions, my patients were becoming dependent upon me to stay well. Yes, I was recommending natural aids and lifestyle changes over conventional treatments but I was not yet addressing the root of their issues.

My goal as a healthcare provider has always been for my patients to become independent by helping them learn to listen to their bodies - eat what they need, sleep as much as they need, exercise as much as they need - to heal. And I've found that by focusing on balancing their hypothalamus that they were able to pay attention to what their bodies really needed and make better choices for themselves.

I hope you enjoy reading The Hypothalamus Handbook. I organized it in a way that you might be able to recognize your symptoms, have a better understanding of your health issues and actually create a therapeutic plan of action. I also organized this book in a way that your healthcare provider can find what they need backed up by references to help you heal.

This book has been a long time coming. Yet it's only been in the last 10 years that research is starting to support the work I've been doing with my patients for over three decades.

Being a pioneer in hypothalamus healing has not been easy, but it's been very rewarding. I've been honored to witness infertile patients finally get pregnant, complicated menopause patients get control of their symptoms and age gracefully, people suffering from chronic fatigue and fibromyalgia be able to have an active lifestyle again, people with multiple endocrinopathies able to wean off hormone replacement therapy as their glands start to function again, people with mood disorders, learning disabilities, neurological dysfunctions finally balance their brain chemistry, people with metabolic disorders stop struggling to get their weight, blood sugar and systemic inflammation under control and finally live their best lives.

We may continue to be bombarded by toxins and infectious agents and our food may not be as nourishing as it needs to be, yet with the proper hypothalamus support, our bodies can clear toxins, fight off infection, control mutations as our DNA begins encoding for healthy metabolism, healthy cellular function, healthy hormone and neurotransmitter metabolism, optimized immune function, and proper detoxification.

With a properly functioning hypothalamus, you can live your best life with optimal health - physically, mentally, emotionally, even energetically because when your hormones sing your DNA dances. Your hypothalamus is the maestro of the symphony of hormones, neurotransmitters, and immune factors to help you survive and more so thrive.

Part One

Meet Your Hypothalamus

Chapter 1

The Boss of Your Body

Albert came to me anxious, tired, unable to sleep and overweight. This 46 year old man had seen seven other healthcare providers, was taking a half dozen prescription meds, and at least a dozen supplements. He had consulted with functional medical specialists who ran a myriad of tests, put him through various detoxification protocols and added more supplements. His conventional doctors couldn't find anything wrong in his bloodwork. They even referred him for psychotherapy. Over the past ten years, Albert had tried everything but nothing was working.

I looked over his test results, took an in-depth history, even probing into his childhood, did a thorough physical exam, and told him, "No one has addressed the root cause of your issue."

"What is it?"

"Your hypothalamus isn't happy."

"My what...?"

Your hypothalamus is the best kept secret in medicine.

Your hypothalamus is a tiny organ in the middle of your brain. And it can't be accessed. We can see it on imaging, but there's no standard way to measure its function. Not by blood work or saliva testing or urine testing.

So how do we know what's going on with your hypothalamus?

Well, in order to determine hypothalamus dysfunction, a healthcare provider must put all your signs and symptoms together. Symptoms are what you're experiencing that feels out of balance. Signs are what healthcare providers note on your physical exam and in your diagnostic tests.

Oh, yes, there are signs and symptoms of hypothalamic dysfunction. But it may take a medical detective to notice them.

For instance, there are markers in the blood work that are off balance. While we're not able to measure hypothalamic hormones directly, when other hormones are out of balance with one another, it can be a sign of hypothalamus dysfunction.

An experienced medical detective is able to read the body and understand what's going on with the hormones, neurotransmitters and immune factors by eliciting your health narrative, confirming your medical history, and performing a thorough physical exam to help determine hypothalamus dysfunction.

Anything off in your neuro-immune-endocrine system is a good indication that the master controller - your hypothalamus - is not functioning properly.

Think of your hypothalamus as the operating system of your physical computer.

The software applications are the hormones produced by your neuro-immune-endocrine system. If you don't have an operating system, these software programs aren't going to work. Your hypothalamus is the operating system that orchestrates all of the different physiological functions of your body - all the messengers - your hormones, your neurotransmitters, your immune factors.

Your hypothalamus is literally the boss of your body.

Your hypothalamus controls everything - your autonomic nervous system, your memory, emotions, sleep, energy production, all your hormones, your immune function, your appetite and weight, your body temperature, heart rate, blood pressure, salt/water balance, and directs your social, sexual, emotive and learning behaviors. There isn't much that your hypothalamus doesn't control.

I believe the function or malfunction of your hypothalamus underlies everything going on in your body. And the past ten years or so, science has proven what I've seen clinically in my healthcare practice. Your hypothalamus is at the root of many diseases.

I first became interested in the hypothalamus twenty-five years ago. After ten years working in conventional medicine, I had opened my own integrative practice, Full Circle Family Health, in July 1997. I wanted more time with my patients to really figure out what was going on with them. I didn't want to be forced to follow a one size fits all protocol typical in conventional medical practices. I wanted to be able to offer my patients more than prescription drugs. I wanted to explore botanicals, bioidentical hormones, nutritional and alternative options as part of the therapeutic plans I would develop with my patients. I desired the freedom to educate my patients on how their bodies work and what they needed to do to achieve balance.

I really wanted to be able to use functional medicine practices and develop a deeper understanding of the neuro-immune-endocrine system. My intention was to learn everything I could possibly learn about the neuro-immune-endocrine system and how to help my patients achieve optimal health physically, mentally and spiritually. And I wanted them to be able to learn how to heal themselves.

The universe complied by sending me the sickest people you could imagine. In medicine, we call these people train wrecks because they have multiple conditions, they've seen multiple specialists, and they're still not well. These patients came to me with loads of prescription drugs and supplements yet were still struggling with their health issues. They wanted to switch from their conventional treatments, like synthetic drugs and hormones, to more natural treatments. Yet they were leaving my office with a horrendous amount of supplementation. And still dependent on me to adjust their regimens.

Honestly, I couldn't have taken all that I was sending them home with. And I felt like I was missing something. I wasn't truly getting to the root of their issues.

Many of these patients presented with similar issues. Weight problems. Sleeping issues. Feeling depressed or anxious or both. Signs of low thyroid function, although bloodwork didn't always support clinical hypothyroidism. Signs of adrenal dysfunction, mostly adrenal insufficiency, but not classic Addison's disease. Gut issues. Detox issues. They had a lot of things going on. So I started doing research trying to uncover a core reason for so much dysfunction. Except search engines were not great for medical research back in the late 90's.

That's when I came across a Scientific American magazine and found a study on white mice which had a lot of the same symptoms my patients did. When the scientists sacrificed the mice, they discovered that the hypothalamus wasn't making enough of a particular hormone which controlled all the dysfunction we were seeing in the mice and I believed...my patients.

If I could focus on the hypothalamus, maybe I wouldn't have to give my patients so much stuff - natural albeit but a lot to take and all of which needed my expertise to guide them. I truly didn't want them dependent on me but desired to help them heal their root issue.

Healing their hypothalamus turned out to be the key.

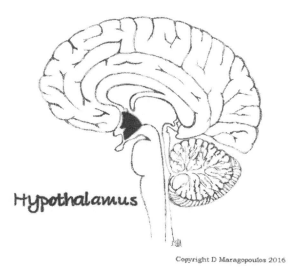

Hypothalamus

Copyright D Maragopoulos 2016

Where is your hypothalamus?

Your hypothalamus sits directly above the brainstem and below the thalamus. Your pea sized pituitary gland hangs from your hypothalamus. Your entire brain weighs about 1400 grams. Your hypothalamus only weighs four grams (about the size of an almond).

Unlike the rest of your brain, your hypothalamus is not protected by the blood brain barrier. A healthy blood brain barrier protects your brain from toxins and infections. Yet the hypothalamus is not protected which is actually a biological imperative. Your hypothalamus reads what's going on in your bloodstream, what nutrients you're getting, how much electrolytes and blood cells are available, what toxins you're being exposed to, what micro-organisms have invaded, what's happening with all your hormones, what's happening in your gut especially your microbiome, and what's happening with your cytokines, the immune factors that help your body protect itself.

Your hypothalamus maintains homeostasis - perfect body balance. And it's programmed for you to survive. Since your hypothalamus is not protected by the blood brain barrier it is very amenable to nutrients.

What does your hypothalamus do?

Your hypothalamus is the maestro of your entire symphony of hormones, neurotransmitters and immune factors. Think of your hypothalamus as the CEO of your body. It orchestrates all major body systems:

- reproduction
- metabolism
- detoxification
- blood pressure and heart rate
- circadian rhythm
- sleep and awareness
- weight set point
- food intake - hunger and satiety
- glucose metabolism
- fluid balance
- temperature regulation
- energy production

- immune function

- autonomic nervous system

- stress response

- emotional expression

- aggression

- memory

- moods

- sexual arousal

Your hypothalamus is at the top of the neuromuscular control of your central nervous system. Your hypothalamus integrates both internal body stimulus as well as external environmental information about your state of well being. Throughout your entire lifespan, your hypothalamus orchestrates physiology to maintain homeostasis or balance.

Your hypothalamus receives sensory and emotional information from your brain. The spinal cord directly communicates pain and temperature information to your hypothalamus. Your hypothalamus integrates all the stimulus it receives and activates patterns of action in your brain and sends signals down your spine to your muscles to produce behaviors.

Your hypothalamus does not only control hormone production by your gonads, your thyroid, your adrenals, your pancreas, your pituitary gland and your pineal gland, it also controls your motor function and your behavior.

Your hypothalamus is made up of large nerve cells called nuclei. Unlike the nuclei in the rest of your brain, the nuclei of the hypothalamus produce hormones. The hypothalamic nuclei are responsible for receiving information and directing action.

In the anterior or front of the hypothalamus, there are five nuclei. In the middle of the hypothalamus, there are four nuclei. And in the posterior or back of the hypothalamus, there are two major nuclei.

Eleven nerve cells control everything in your body!

Your hypothalamus regulates your neuro-immune-endocrine system. These three systems produce biochemical messengers that direct all your body functions. And your hypothalamus is the maestro of it all.

Your hypothalamus orchestrates your endocrine system.

So far science has identified over 50 hormones. Hormones are produced by many organs, including your gut, your fat cells, your kidneys, your parathyroid. The most well known hormones are produced by your endocrine system.

Different from exocrine glands like your salivary glands which produce enzymes that work locally on food in your mouth, endocrine glands produce hormones that work distantly in the body, traveling through the bloodstream to enter cells via receptor sites and do their work.

Your seven endocrine glands are:

1. **Gonads** - Ovaries produce estrogen, progesterone and testosterone. Testes produce testosterone.

2. **Pancreas** - Your pancreas lies to the left and under your stomach. Your pancreas is both an exocrine gland producing digestive enzymes, but also an endocrine gland producing insulin and glucagon.

3. **Adrenals** - Your adrenal glands sit on top of your kidneys and produce adrenaline, pregnenolone, DHEA, cortisol and aldosterone.

4. **Thymus** - Your thymus lies just above your heart. Your thymus produces and releases several hormones. Thymopoietin fuels the production of T-cells and tells the pituitary gland to release hormones. Thymosin and thymulin help make specialized types of T-cells. Thymic humoral factor keeps your immune system working properly.

5. **Thyroid** - Your thyroid lies at the base of your throat and produces thyroxine (T_4) which gets converted into its active form triiodothyronine (T_3). Behind your thyroid are the parathyroid glands which produce parathyroid hormone that regulates calcium.

6. **Pituitary** - Your pituitary gland lies beneath your hypothalamus. Under the direction of your hypothalamus, your pituitary gland acts as middle manager producing stimulating hormones to activate the lower endocrine glands - gonads, adrenals, thyroid. Your pituitary gland also produces growth hormone and stores and releases the hypothalamus hormones - prolactin and oxytocin.

7. **Pineal** - Your pineal gland lies in the middle of your brain. Your pineal gland produces melatonin.

In part two, I will explain what your hormones do in relation to real case studies.

Your hypothalamus orchestrates your neurological system.

Your hypothalamus orchestrates all hormonal type messengers including neurotransmitters. Your nerves produce neurotransmitters to communicate with each other. There are more than 100 neurotransmitters made by your nervous system; some of the most important are acetylcholine, norepinephrine, dopamine, gamma-aminobutyric acid (GABA), glutamate, serotonin, and histamine.

Neurotransmitters are produced by your brain, your heart and your gut.

If I had to put them in order by importance for your survival - your heart would be number one, your gut number two, and your brain number three. If there's only so many amino acids to make neurotransmitters like serotonin or dopamine, they're going to go to the heart first, then the gut and then the brain so you can survive. So in order to survive at the biochemical level, you may feel depressed or anxious.

Your hypothalamus controls your:

Autonomic nervous system. Your autonomic nervous system (ANS) is not under your conscious control. The ANS has two branches - the sympathetic and parasympathetic. The sympathetic nervous system produces excitatory neurotransmitters. The parasympathetic nervous system produces calming neurotransmitters.

Through the autonomic nervous system, your hypothalamus stimulates smooth muscle which lines your blood vessels, stomach and intestines and receives sensory information from these areas. That's how your hypothalamus controls your heart rate and blood pressure, the passage of food through your intestinal tract, your bladder contractions as well as other visceral organs.

Emotional responses. Your hypothalamus lies at the center of the emotional part of your brain called the limbic system. Your hypothalamus is the brain's intermediary for translating emotion into physical response. Physical signs of fear or excitement, like a racing heart, shallow breathing, even a clenching gut feeling all originate in your hypothalamus.

Motivational behavior. Your hypothalamus controls rewarding behavior. That's because your hypothalamus is the main producer of dopamine - the reward neurotransmitter. Your hypothalamus influences your motivation to eat, to have sex, to act.

Formation of memory. Your hypothalamus directly stimulates memory updates as well as secondary behaviors through motivational dopamine pathways and arousal autonomic nervous system pathways to initiate and reinforce learning. Your hypothalamus receives input from your brain's memory processing center helping you associate memory with emotion. That's why highly emotional events are more memorable.

Your hypothalamus orchestrates your immune system.

Your immune system's job is to protect you. Your immune system includes your thymus which is the endocrine gland right over your heart that programs your white blood cells. Your immune system also includes your lymph nodes, appendix, tonsils and adenoids, spleen, and bone marrow which produces blood cells.

Your white blood cells act like soldiers patrolling your tissues and protecting you from invasion. White blood cells called lymphocytes are produced in the bone marrow and are called B-cells. These soldiers go to the thymus which acts like boot camp to program the white blood cells. Once programmed these lymphocytes are called T-cells.

Your thymus produces hormones that program your white blood cells to know the difference between you and other. If they do not get programmed properly, your white blood cells attack you which is known as autoimmunity.

Whatever you've been exposed to in the past, like childhood chickenpox, your thymus remembers. When you're young, your T-cells remember the varicella virus which causes chicken pox to protect you from another out-break. When you're middle aged, your T-cells can begin to forget varicella virus, so exposure to a child with chicken pox can induce another varicella reaction called shingles. By the time women are postmenopausal and men are in their sixties, the thymus isn't doing as good a job because it's been shrinking over the years.

Your thymus is largest in early childhood as it actively receives hormonal messages called cytokines from the foraging white blood cells about the environment and then programs lymphocytes accordingly. Over the years, the thymus naturally shrinks until by the seventh or eighth decade it's barely functioning which is why cancer is much more prevalent with age.

When X-rays were first developed, doctors were alarmed by the huge size of the thymus in children and routinely irradiated them. These children developed autoimmune diseases and cancer very early in life. Your thymus is a vital endocrine gland.

Your immune system produces hormones called cytokines. Two hundred cytokines have been identified so far. Your hypothalamus directly affects your immune system through circadian hormones.

I use the term hormone to refer to all biochemical messengers that use receptor sites to enter cells - neurotransmitters, cytokines, and hormones. The neuro-immune-endocrine system produces these messengers and your hypothalamus orchestrates it all.

Your hypothalamus is the maestro of your symphony of hormones. Wisely supporting your hypothalamus helps keep all your Hormones in Harmony®.

Chapter 2

The Root of All Health Issues

Judy came to me with weight loss, food sensitivities, osteoporosis, muscle mass loss, blood sugar issues and very itchy skin. She'd been suffering with food sensitivities and blood sugar issues for years.

She had consulted with specialists in endocrinology, internal medicine, functional medicine, yet no one could figure out why she was so out of balance. And unfortunately, she kept losing more weight, more muscle mass, more bone density.

Judy's adrenals were producing too much cortisol which created a resultant flux in her blood sugar. The high cortisol destroyed the epithelial lining of her intestine which caused a lot of her food issues.

But in spite of colon healing measures, blood sugar stabilizing medications, supplements and diet changes, Judy couldn't get in balance. No one was addressing her hypothalamus.

The hypothalamus produces hormones that regulate glucose metabolism. The hypothalamus also regulates the stress response and adrenal production of cortisol.

The hypothalamus regulates digestion, absorption of nutrients, and body fat storage. So until we started focusing on Judy's hypothalamus, balancing it with nutraceuticals and lifestyle changes, did she finally get better, was able to tolerate many more foods, keep her blood sugar stable and gain back lean body mass.

If your hypothalamus is so important why is it ignored?

Because it's difficult to determine hypothalamus function. You can't measure the hormones from the hypothalamus to definitively diagnose hypothalamic dysfunction. You need a medical detective to figure it out.

Most healthcare providers practice downstream medicine. Whether they're conventional or functional, complementary or integrative, most healthcare providers work hard to help relieve your symptoms. Yet they do not often get to the root of your health issues. Yes, their pharmaceuticals, botanicals, or homeopathics may help relieve your symptoms, but without digging deep into your history, looking closely at your lifestyle choices, taking your genetics into account, they will not be addressing the core problem.

Let's say you have Lyme disease. Your healthcare provider will give you antimicrobials, either antibiotics or botanicals to kill the bug. And they may give you some supplements to help heal up your neurological system.

But what they don't do is get to the core issue. Yes, you got bitten by a tick which infected you with Borrelia bacterium, but why did you get Lyme disease in the first place? Why didn't your immune system fight it off in the beginning? Why did your body allow the bacterium to multiply and attack your nervous system, your immune system, your gut?

Because your hypothalamus is out of balance. If your hypothalamus is in balance, your immune system functions pristinely and protects you. That doesn't mean you're not going to catch viruses, but you fight them off quickly.

One of the things that I noticed by supporting my hypothalamus for over 20 years is that oftentimes I will sense that I've been exposed to something. I'll walk into a patient's room who has some kind of an upper respiratory infection. First, I embrace the mindset that 'this is not my bug' before I go in and probably breathe in the virus. Even if I feel tickling in my throat, my immune system fights it off immediately. My patients who work with small children tell me that after supporting their hypothalamus for a few months, they don't get sick nearly as often. And we all know what Petri dishes little kids are.

Upstream Medicine

Focusing on the root issue and treating the hypothalamus is upstream medicine. Of course I provide my patients with immediate symptom relief, but if I don't focus on treating their hypothalamus, they will be dependent on me for constant symptom relief.

Going through the change of life - menopause or andropause for men - stimulates hypothalamic dysfunction. When your sex steroids bottom out, your hypothalamus becomes dysfunctional. And you don't have to be middle age to experience hot flashes, brain fog, low libido, aging skin, loss of lean body mass from low sex hormones. Young men with hypogonadism, which means they're not producing enough testosterone and young women with premature ovarian failure, which means they're running out of eggs and sex hormones before 35 years of age, suffer from hypothalamic dysfunction.

Polycystic ovary syndrome is almost always rooted in hypothalamic dysfunction. Infertility and irregular periods often indicate problems in the hypothalamus. Thyroid issues, either hyperthyroidism - too much thyroid hormone - or hypothyroidism - too little thyroid hormone - often have a central component meaning the hypothalamus is involved. Most adrenal issues are caused by an inefficient hypothalamic-pituitary-adrenal (HPA) axis.

Many gut issues are rooted in hypothalamic dysfunction. Your hypothalamus and your gut are connected. It's the hypothalamus that actually controls hunger hormones, detoxification pathways, and nutrient absorption.

Mood disorders - anxiety and depression - are rooted in hypothalamic dysfunction. Learning disabilities including autism have been shown to involve hypothalamus dysfunction. Eating disorders like anorexia and bulimia have been shown to shrink the hypothalamus. Chronic depression and bipolar conditions do too.

Addictions are rooted in the hypothalamus. That's because addictions are dopamine driven and dopamine is controlled by the hypothalamus.

Metabolic syndrome, characterized by high blood pressure, insulin resistance, high cholesterol, is an inflammatory condition that is rooted in the hypothalamus and causes more hypothalamic dysfunction. Downstream medicine treats metabolic syndrome with multiple drugs - antihypertensives, statins, antidiabetic medications - all of which are appropriate with lifestyle management yet without practicing upstream medicine and treating the inflamed hypothalamus - the patient is dependent on pharmaceuticals for life.

Autoimmune disorders are also rooted in hypothalamic dysfunction. Your hypothalamus produces prolactin which controls the immune system. Autoimmunity often affects pituitary production of stimulating hormones. Hypopituitaryism is a condition where you don't make enough pituitary hormones so your lower endocrine glands make insufficient amounts of sex hormones, thyroid hormone and adrenal hormones. You become dependent for life on total hormone replacement therapy, unless you heal your hypothalamus. Remember your pituitary is the middle manager, the boss of your body is your hypothalamus.

Why are Hypothalamic hormones so important?

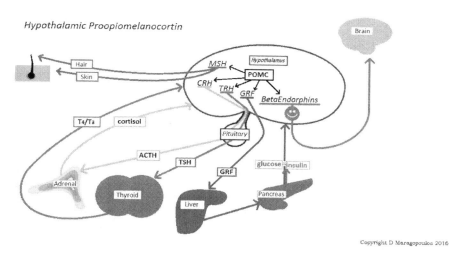

Hypothalamic Proopiomelanocortin

Copyright D Maragopoulos 2016

Without hypothalamic hormones, you wouldn't survive.

Pro-opiomelanocortin (POMC) is a great example of how involved your hypothalamus is in so many vital systems.

POMC is a huge 241 amino acid molecule that gets broken down into cortico releasing hormone (CRH), which stimulates the pituitary to release adrenocorticotrophic hormone (ACTH). ACTH stimulates your adrenals to produce cortisol.

The adrenals, like the thyroid, are in a negative feedback system with the hypothalamus and pituitary gland. If cortisol's high, ACTH is low and back and forth in a seesaw effect.

POMC breaks down to lipotropin which stimulates your liver to release fat. Your hypothalamus is so sensitive to blood glucose levels that it insures your brain and vital organs get enough glucose to create cellular energy.

POMC breaks down to melanocyte stimulating hormone (MSH), which gives you color to your skin and hair, but also controls your day/night cycles and your metabolism.

What's left over of the POMC hormone becomes beta endorphins. Endorphins are your feel good neurotransmitters.

POMC is one hypothalamic hormone that controls your stress response, your glucose metabolism, your circadian rhythm and your moods.

POMC controls your appetite and energy expenditure. POMC neurons in the arcuate nucleus of the hypothalamus are activated by energy surplus and inhibited by energy deficit. When activated, POMC cells inhibit food intake and facilitate weight loss. Decreased activity in POMC cells is associated with increased food intake and obesity.

While POMC is made in the arcuate nucleus, cortico releasing hormone is stored and released by the paraventricular nucleus which also makes thyroid releasing hormone. If your adrenal glands are off, it's going to throw your thyroid and glucose metabolism off. Plus you may not be as happy as you used to be. All of this is controlled by just one hypothalamic hormone.

And that's why I look at the lower endocrine glands that I can measure to give me a gist of what's going on in the hypothalamus. It helps me determine if your hypothalamus is actually out of balance.

Your hypothalamus and your DNA

Your hypothalamus is at the center of your pyramid of health.

Hormones in Harmony®

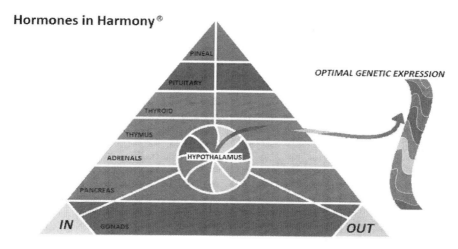

Copyright D Marangopoulos 2016

The base of the pyramid is your sex steroid production. The next level is how much insulin your pancreas produces to get glucose into the cells. Your adrenal function makes up the third level. Your thymus protects you at the fourth level and at the fifth level your thyroid regulates your metabolism. At the sixth level, your pituitary gland acts as middle manager and releases its own hormones. Your pineal gland at the top must make melatonin so you can sleep and rejuvenate.

The cornerstones of your pyramid of health are what you're eating and what you're getting out including toxins and energy production. Your hypothalamus is very sensitive to what you're putting into your body. If you're not giving it the nutrients it needs, it's not going to be able to help you orchestrate your hormones in the most pristine way.

That's why diet and proper supplementation is really important. And if you're not detoxifying properly - getting waste out of the body through cellular detoxification, as well as liver and kidney detoxification, your hypothalamus cannot function properly. Remember your hypothalamus is not protected by the blood brain barrier, so it's very sensitive to how toxic you are. If you're toxic, your hypothalamus is going to slow your metabolism down so you don't become poisoned by your own cellular waste.

It's not uncommon for someone with a weight issue or fatigue to be toxic. If they're toxic, their hypothalamus goes into survival mode so that it can spend energy, nutrients and resources on trying to detox.

Your hypothalamus is at the center of your pyramid of health. All hormonal messengers through the orchestration of the hypothalamus direct your genetic expression. You have millions of potential genes that can be expressed so you can achieve optimal health. You are not stuck with what you're born with. Your DNA is not cast in stone.

You have much more unexpressed genetics than genes that are expressed - meaning activated to form you, your body tissues, your enzymes, your hormones, your neurotransmitters, your immune cytokines - much more potential than you realize.

But what if you have "bad" genes - familial heart disease or cancer? Can you change that genetic expression? Or are you destined to get the same diseases that your family has suffered from?

You can change your genetic expression. If your hypothalamus is functioning optimally and directing healthy balanced hormones, your DNA can shift from expressing disease to healing. It's called epigenetics - the ability for DNA to change its expression throughout a person's life.

Your lifestyle choices - what you eat, how active you are, how much sleep you get, what you believe - influences your genetic expression. Your DNA is not cast in stone but is malleable like wet clay according to the choices you make that affect your hypothalamus.

Since your hypothalamus helps regulate genetic expression, if you desire optimal health, you need to focus healing therapies on your optimizing hypothalamic function.

Chapter 3

When Your Hypothalamus Isn't Happy

When your hypothalamus isn't happy, it's called hypothalamus dysfunction.

Hypothalamus dysfunction is defined as insufficient production of hypothalamic hormones. Without adequate hypothalamus hormones, pituitary function is diminished. Poor hypothalamus function affects all lower endocrine glands - thyroid, adrenals, ovaries, testes, pancreas as well as your pineal gland.

Hypothalamus dysfunction affects brain function, immune function, digestion, metabolism and circadian rhythm. Hypothalamus dysfunction affects thermoregulation, appetite, energy, mood and memory.

While the majority of hypothalamic dysfunction affects the HPA axis which influences adrenal function, all aspects of hypothalamus function can be affected. Vasopressin and oxytocin production is suppressed. Dopamine levels fall, prolactin rises. Sex hormones become imbalanced. Thyroid function is affected. Your sleep is disturbed. Your energy is low. Your moods and memory are affected.

Since your hypothalamus controls every vital system of your body, when it's not functioning properly everything is affected.

How prevalent is hypothalamus dysfunction?

Well, it's more common than most people realize. If you've ever had a traumatic brain injury then there's up to 80% likelihood you may have hypothalamus dysfunction. If you're a woman who does not have periods, there's a 35% chance your secondary amenorrhea is caused by hypothalamus dysfunction. If you survived childhood cancer, there's a 40% chance you have hypothalamus dysfunction. And if you're female, you have twice the likelihood your hypothalamus is dysfunctional following brain injury.

Symptoms of hypothalamic dysfunction

Symptoms of hypothalamic dysfunction are varied according to what part of the hypothalamus is damaged and may include:

- Fatigue
- Temperature dysregulation - cold all the time, hot flashes, night sweats, fevers
- Appetite changes - anorexia or hyperphagia
- Weight loss or weight gain with or without changes in appetite
- Changes in sleep - trouble falling asleep or staying asleep
- Pain - especially trigger point tenderness
- Mood disorders - anxiety, depression
- Libido issues
- High blood pressure or low blood pressure

- Water retention
- Dehydration
- Excessive thirst
- Excessive urination
- Irritable bowel with maldigestion, malabsorption, constipation, diarrhea
- Amenorrhea
- Irregular periods
- Infertility
- Osteoporosis
- Delayed puberty
- Sarcopenia - loss of muscle
- Weakness
- Premature aging
- Sympathetic symptoms - palpitations, panic attacks, sweating, insomnia
- Parasympathetic symptoms - delayed digestion, arrhythmias, somnolence
- Lack of motivation
- Inability to bond with others
- Maladaptive stress response
- Skin rashes, acne, eczema

What causes Hypothalamus Dysfunction?

Most cases of hypothalamus dysfunction are caused by trauma. Although I see many patients with hypothalamus dysfunction with no history of brain injury, they often have a history of malnutrition, infections, or toxic exposures. Sometimes it's chronic stress or a single traumatic event.

Here are the most common causes of hypothalamus dysfunction:

- Brain surgery
- Traumatic brain injury
- Brain tumors
- Radiation
- Chemotherapy
- Nutritional deficiencies
- Nutritional excess -high saturated fats, high glycemic index carbohydrates
- Brain aneurysms
- Genetic disorders (Prader-Willi syndrome, Kallmann syndrome)
- Infections (EBV, Lyme, TB, covid)
- Inflammatory diseases (multiple sclerosis, neurosarcoidosis)
- Heat stroke
- Chronic stress

More and more often, I see cases of hypothalamus dysfunction from chronic stress. Stress wreaks havoc on your hormones setting off a cascade of hypothalamic symptoms.

So what happens if your hypothalamus is dysfunctional?

Most hormonal imbalances, immune issues, neurological disorders and chronic illnesses are rooted in hypothalamus dysfunction.

Hypothalamus dysfunction plays a role in many health issues

Name of Condition	Connection to Hypothalamus
Acromegaly and pituitary gigantism	Rare disorders of growth due to excessive release of growth hormone from your pituitary gland which is controlled by your hypothalamus.
Addictions	Your hypothalamus is often at the root of addictive behaviors. Cocaine addiction has recently been associated with hypothalamic dysfunction.
Aging	Studios show that hypothalamic micro inflammation initiates cellular aging. Hypothalamic microinflammation
Amenorrhea	The absence of a period for more than three months in people assigned female at birth (AFAB) who previously had regular periods or more than six months in people AFAB who have irregular menstruation. The most common cause of this condition is hypothalamic dysfunction.
Autoimmunity	Your hypothalamus regulates your immune function. Studies show that hypothalamus dysfunction is often at the root of autoimmune conditions.
Cardiovascular disease	Patients with hypothalamic-pituitary disease are known to have increased cardiovascular risk
Central hypothyroidism	A rare disorder that occurs due to both hypothalamic and pituitary disorders. The most common cause is a pituitary tumor such as a pituitary adenoma.
Central Obesity	Studies have shown that obese people with thyroid symptoms often have hypothalamic dysfunction. Dysfunctional insulin and leptin receptors within the hypothalamus may have a role in hypothalamic obesity. Diets with abundant saturated tatty acids cause mitochondria dysfunction and inflammatory response in the hypothalamus, producing hypothalamic dysfunction, which promotes obesity. Activation of hypothalamic inflammatory pathways results in the uncoupling or caloric intake and energy expenditure, fostering overeating and further weight gain.
CFS/Myalgic Encephalitis	Your hypothalamus controls mitochondrial energy output and cellular metabolism. Hypothalamus dysfunction is often at the root or chronic fatique syndrome now known as myalgic encephalitis
Diabetes insipidus	When your hypothalamus doesn't produce and release enough vasopressin, your kidneys lose too much water which results in excessive urination and thirst.
Diabetes/insulin resistance	Hypothalamic inflammation links central insulin resistance to diabetes. Hypothalamic regulation of feeding body weight, and glucose homeostasis is mediated by multiple signaling pathways including insulin signaling.
Hyperprolactinemia	A decrease in hypothalamic dopamine levels causes an increase in prolactin levels. Causes may include a tumor or damage to nerve cells in the hypothalamus.
Hypothalamic-pituitary disorders	Because of the close interactions between your hypothalamus and pituitary gland, conditions that affect either are often caused by hypothalamus dysfunction.

Hypothalamus dysfunction plays a role in many health issues

Name of Condition	Connection to Hypothalamus
Hypopituitarism	When your pituitary gland does not make enough stimulating hormones or its own hormones. Damage to your hypothalamus can cause hypopituitarism.
Insomnia	Your hypothalamus controls your day night cycles and is at the root of most sleep disorders including sleep apnea.
Kallmann Syndrome	Has a genetic link to hypothalamic disease, causing such hypothalamic problems in children as delayed or no puberty.
Mood Disorders	Has a genetic link to hypothalamic disease, causing such hypothalamic problems in children as delayed or no puberty.
Pain	Studies show that your hypothalamus regulates pain sensation and hypothalamus dysfunction is often at the root of chronic pain disorders like fibromyalgia.
Prader-Willi Syndrome	An inherited disorder which causes your hypothalamus not to recognize the sensation that you're full when you're eating, resulting in a constant urge to eat and morbid obesity.
Reproductive issues/Infertility	Your hypothalamus regulates reproduction including the timing of puberty, menstrual periods, fertility, menopause and andropause.
Syndrome of inappropriate antidiuretic hormone	Elevated hypothalamic antidiuretic hormone level can be caused by stroke, hemorrhage, infection, trauma cancer and certain medications.

New studies on cell aging show that aging begins in the hypothalamus. In every cell of your body exists a network of membranous tubules that carry on the work instructed by your DNA. This vital network is called the endoplasmic reticulum (ER). The ER folds proteins to create new you.

The ER is the major site of protein synthesis and transport to make tissues and biochemicals. The ER synthesizes lipids (fats) and steroids (hormones). The ER metabolizes carbohydrates for mitochondrial energy production. The ER stores calcium which is vital for extracellular transport, muscle cell contraction, neurotransmitter release and fertilization.

The endoplasmic reticulum is dependent upon healthy cell membrane function. Your cell membrane transports vital nutrients into the cell and waste products out. When your cell membrane becomes damaged by malnutrition, infections or toxins, it affects all cell function but especially the ER.

Endoplasmic reticulum stress refers to physiological or pathological states in which proteins are unfolded or misfolded in the ER. Hypothalamic ER stress plays a critical role in mediating neuroinflammation and neuronal injury, as well as regulating food intake, energy expenditure, and body weight.

When your ER can no longer adequately fold proteins, your cells die. ER stress can be induced by environmental factors: glucose deprivation/caloric restriction, lipid composition and concentration inside and outside of your cells, toxins like heavy metals, certain drugs, pesticides, herbicides, and even toxic lipids. Which is why it's so important to eat the right fats.

Obesity can cause ER stress. Maternal obesity induced ER stress can cause metabolic issues in the fetus and prevent normal hypothalamus development.

The health of your cells affects hypothalamus function and your hypothalamus affects cellular health and function.

How does your healthcare provider determine you have hypothalamus dysfunction?

It's not easy. Hypothalamus dysfunction is often a diagnosis of exclusion. We've ruled out everything else and determine it must be your hypothalamus that's at the root of your issues.

Yes, there are signs - in your body and lab studies. Yet it may take a medical detective to uncover hypothalamus dysfunction.

For example, many people with hypothyroid symptoms will have a normal thyroid blood panel - yet they suffer from fatigue, constipation, cold extremities, hair loss, menstrual irregularities, weight gain. Studies show that most of these patients are treated as malingering - which means they're believed to be complaining about nothing.

But that's not the case. These patients probably have hypothalamic dysfunction and their thyroid function is not yet affected. Wouldn't it be great if they could get relief sooner?

In over thirty years of treating hypothalamus dysfunction, I have found that it's necessary to do a complete history and physical as well as get appropriate lab studies.

Here's what I do:

First, I get a thorough history on my patients by asking these questions:

- What's your most aggravating symptom?
- What other symptoms are you experiencing?
- When did your symptoms begin?
- What have you tried to treat these symptoms? Has anything worked?
- Was there a significant stressor that preceded your illness? What are the major stressors in your life now? In the past? Is there a history of abuse - emotional, physical, or sexual?
- What diagnoses have you been given?
- What tests have been run?
- What medications are you taking? Why and for how long?
- What supplements are you taking? Why and for how long?
- How was your health as a child?
- How was your mother's health when she was pregnant with you? Was she obese?
- Did you experience childhood trauma? Divorce? Abuse of parent or self? Substance abuse in the household? Chronic illness of caretakers? Food insecurity or shelter insecurity?
- Have you ever had a traumatic brain injury?

- Have you had Epstein Barr virus, tuberculosis, Lyme, and/or Covid?

- Have you been diagnosed with myalgic encephalomyelitis/chronic fatigue syndrome or fibromyalgia?

- Do you now have or have you in the past had a high exposure to toxins? Heavy metals? Pesticides? Herbicides? Chemotherapy?

- Does anyone in your family have similar health problems?

- How long does family typically live? What do members of your family die from?

- How much sleep do you get? Is it interrupted? Do you need sleep aids? Do you remember your dreams? Do you wake up refreshed?

- How is your energy? Do you have lulls during the day? When is your energy the highest?

- What's your diet like? How much protein do you consume daily? How much fat? What kind of carbs do you eat? How many fruits do you get daily? How many vegetables and what types? What do you crave?

- How's your appetite? Do you eat emotionally?

- Do any foods cause issues for you? What issues - gastrointestinal, skin, sinus, mood changes?

- How much water, caffeine, alcohol, sweetened or artificially sweetened beverages do you drink daily?

- Do you use recreational substances? Have you had an issue of abusing alcohol, pain medications, or stimulants?

- Women, at what age did you start menstruating? What is/was your cycle length? Do you suffer from extreme cramps, breast tenderness, moodiness, or menstrual migraines? How many times have you been pregnant? How did you feel during your pregnancies? How many live births? Any miscarriages? Any problems with infertility? If so, what treatments were you given?

- Men, at what age did you experience nocturnal emissions (wet dreams)? When did you reach your adult height? Do you have regular morning erections? Do you have any problems with impotency? Have you ever impregnated a woman?

- What is your main healing goal?

- What are you willing to do to achieve this goal?

- Do you believe you can heal?

Then I do a thorough physical exam. I note:

- Body habitus - Is my patient endomorphic (thin), mesomorphic (muscular) or ectomorphic (excess body fat)?

- Distribution of body fat - apple shaped (cortisol driven/insulin resistant), pear shaped (estrogen dominant)

- Distribution of muscle - noting deltoid formation in men (flat posterior deltoids are a sign of androgen deficiency)

- Skin - signs of aging, dark areas (melasma on face, dark velvety skin in folds - acanthosis nigricans) or loss of pigment (vitiligo or small depigmented spots on extremities indicates estrogen deficiency), any rashes or acne

- Hair distribution - loss of pubic hair (low adrenal androgens), loss of body hair, thinning eyebrows, loss of outer third of eyebrows (low thyroid), hirsutism or male pattern hair in a female (high androgens), loss of head hair (diffuse - low estrogen/low thyroid vs thinning at temples and crown - high androgens)

- Cardiovascular - checking heart rate and rhythm, carotid bruits, pulses, edema

- Breast exam both male and female checking for masses and nipple discharge and teaching the patient how to examine themselves and what they're looking for

- Abdomen - checking for hepatosplenomegaly, abdominal masses or tenderness

- Thyroid - size, shape, nodularity, tenderness (if enlarged may indicate autoimmune thyroiditis)

- Female pelvic exam - uterine fibroids, ovarian masses

- Male genital exam - inguinal hernias, testicular size and masses

- Rectal exam - if over 40 - checking for masses and occult blood, and in men, checking size and texture of prostate

As you can see the evaluation is pretty extensive.

Next I order appropriate lab studies. First of all, I do bloodwork.

I used to do 24 hour urine and salivary testing along with bloodwork but I have found that it's no longer necessary. In my intuitive medical detective assessment of my hormonally challenged patients, I use bloodwork to support my findings.

In terms of measuring individual hormones, bloodwork is not always accurate. Your hormones are active at the tissue level not in the bloodstream. Measuring hormones in bloodwork is like trying to get a population count of people on the freeways in Los Angeles which is dependent upon which freeway, what time of day, what day of the week you're measuring. Hormones follow circadian patterns and, in women, monthly cycles, so an individual hormone blood test is just a snapshot, not reflective of hormone function or even true endocrine gland production.

What I'm looking for is a comparison of some hormone levels, mostly pituitary hormones and other blood markers that may indicate hypothalamic function.

Your healthcare provider may not interpret the bloodwork in the same way that I do. Oftentimes, you're not alerted that anything is off unless your bloodwork falls out of the normal ranges. Laboratory reference values are based on measuring 1000 or so people of your gender and your age. It's not necessarily your normal.

In the last 30 years since I've been specializing in neuro-immune-endocrinology, hormone levels have drastically changed for both genders. For instance, male testosterone has dropped significantly in the last 20 years. And DHEA levels have dropped significantly for both genders.

Normal in terms of the laboratory reference ranges isn't necessarily optimal for you. So I'm looking at your history, my physical examination of you, as well as your bloodwork to determine your baseline. What you look like hormonally in lab studies compared to what you're experiencing symptomatically. Your pituitary hormones give me a much better marker of sex steroid adequacy for you than measuring your sex hormones individually. And I compare individual hormones to each other to determine hypothalamus function. My favorite triad of bloodwork is looking at your hemoglobin A1C, DHEA-S, and thyroid panel to determine hypothalamic POMC production.

Here's what I look at in your bloodwork:

I do a full **chemistry panel** to check electrolytes as well as liver and kidney health. I need to know if basic detoxification pathways are functioning.

I check glucose metabolism by measuring hemoglobin A1C (**HGBA1C**) which is a protein carried on your red blood cells that is highly sensitive to your blood sugar. HGBA1C is high when your blood glucose has been high over the lifespan of your red blood cells. Better than a fasting glucose,

HGBA1C tells me how high your blood sugar has been over the past two months. High HGBA1C is a marker of insulin resistance and diabetes.

I do a **fasting lipid panel** including subparticle sizes and lipoproteins. Cholesterol is not created equally and total numbers do not reflect particle sizes. Large cholesterol particles are buoyant and protective. Small cholesterol particles are inflammatory and can cause arteriosclerosis. Your steroid hormones are created from large particle low density lipids (LDL). A typical lipid profile does not give me this information.

Think of your total cholesterol filling a plate. At least one third of that plate should be high density lipids (HDL), the rest are LDLs. At least half of your HDL and LDL should be large protective particles. Lipoproteins are how cholesterol is transported. Lipoprotein A reflects how much small density LDL has been floating around in your blood. High levels of lipoprotein A (LPa) reflects an increased risk of heart disease.

Lipid panels typically include triglycerides which are triple sugars on a fat molecule. Your liver packages extra glucose into triglycerides to be stored in your fat cells. Triglycerides are a reflection of how high your blood sugar has been in the past few days.

Another important measure of cardiovascular health is cardio-reactive protein (CRP). CRP measures arterial inflammation. I do a **high sensitivity CRP** on all my patients. If it is elevated in the face of high cholesterol, there is an increased risk of cardiovascular disease. Impaired blood flow to the hypothalamus due to cardiovascular inflammation adversely affects its function.

I measure **serum vitamin D** levels. Vitamin D is a vital prohormone acting to improve cell receptor site function. Hormones must enter cells through cell receptor sites. If vitamin D levels are low, hormone function is affected. Vitamin D is also important in maintaining bone health and promoting healthy immune response.

Then I look at hormones. I start with a **thyroid panel** which is the most reflective of hypothalamic-pituitary axis issues. Your hypothalamus is highly sensitive to active thyroid hormones, working in a negative feedback mechanism to produce thyroid releasing hormone (TRH). Free unbound hormones are active. If free T_4 and free T_3 are low then your hypothalamus produces more TRH to stimulate your pituitary gland to produce thyroid stimulating hormone (TSH). We cannot measure TRH, but we can measure TSH.

Oftentimes I see patients with hypothyroid symptoms but normal levels of thyroid hormones. What I look at is the ratio of **TSH** to **fT4** and **fT3**. Imagine a seesaw. If thyroid hormones are low, then TSH should be high. If thyroid hormones are high, then TSH should be low. If TSH is low normal in the face of low normal active thyroid hormones or visa versa, if TSH is high normal with high normal fT_4 and fT_3 levels, then there is a miscommunication between the hypothalamus, pituitary and thyroid also known as the hypothalamic-pituitary-thyroid axis. This is a clear sign of hypothalamus dysfunction often missed by healthcare providers who are only focusing on individual numbers. If they're all in normal ranges, they believe you're fine. But you're not.

If you're metabolically inactive as reflected by high body fat percentage or fatigue, I may add a **reverse T3** (rT_3). Thyroid hormones are formed by the iodination of thyroglobulin - first as T_4 with four iodine molecules. Then one iodine molecule is removed to create active T_3, but if the wrong iodine molecule is knocked off - it's called rT_3. Reverse T_3 is inactive. When you measure total T_3 levels, you're looking at both active and inactive trioiodothyronine. That's why I mainly look at fT_3 which is the active form of thyroid hormones at the cellular level.

If your thyroid levels are off or I suspect autoimmune thyroiditis, I order thyroid autoantibodies - thyroid peroxidase antibodies (TPO), thyroglobulin antibodies (TBGab), thyroid stimulating immunoglobulin (TSI) which reflects autoimmune hyperthyroidism.

I also look at adrenal function by measuring sulfated dehydroepiandrosterone (**DHEA-S**) which is the activated form of DHEA. DHEA production follows cortisol production. While cortisol releases stored sugar to fuel the stress response, DHEA helps you metabolize protein and fat to repair damage from your fight or flight. Unlike cortisol, DHEA-S can be measured anytime of the day and is not immediately reflective of acute stress.

DHEA-S levels are different according to your age and gender. The highest levels are at the end of adolescence and drop every ten years. Since I've been measuring DHEA-S in all my patients, the normal ranges have dropped significantly. Laboratory norms are determined by the general population and are updated every ten years or so. DHEA-S normal ranges were much higher three decades ago. I believe that's because the amount of stress people are under is contributing to adrenal dysfunction.

If your DHEA-S levels are too low, it may reflect adrenal insufficiency. If DHEA-S levels are too high, it may reflect adrenal hyperactivity. Then I order an 8am cortisol. **Cortisol** has a critical circadian rhythm - high during the day and low at night. But measuring serum cortisol can be tricky as acute stress, like fear of blood draws will immediately elevate it.

If your cortisol is high or low at 8am, I order an ACTH with serum cortisol to be drawn fasting at 8am to check your hypothalamus-pituitary-adrenal axis. Adrenocorticotropic hormone (ACTH) is produced by your pituitary in response to your hypothalamus' production of CRH which responds in a negative feedback with circulating cortisol.

If your DHEA-S levels are out of range, then I also order an **unconjugated DHEA** to measure your adrenal reserve. DHEA production is actually the same in both genders and drops in half after 40 years of age and half again after 70 years of age. I may also order a serum **pregnenelone** which is a precursor hormone to DHEA.

My trifecta of hypothalamic function is to look at your thyroid panel, DHEA-S, and HGBA1C together. These lower endocrine markers reflect hypothalamic POMC function. Even if they're within normal limits, but out of range with one another, I suspect hypothalamus dysfunction.

What about your other hormones - like sex steroids? Well, if you're a menstruating woman, trying to measure your estrogen and progesterone levels is not easy. Your levels of sex steroids change according to the day of your cycle. And the range of normal is very wide. Some women naturally make more estrogen and become symptomatic of estrogen deficiency when their estrogen falls into low normal ranges. Other women make much less estrogen and are symptomatic of estrogen dominance when their estrogen rises to mid or high normal levels. Measuring a woman's follicle stimulating hormone (**FSH**) on day 3-5 of her menstrual cycle (day one is the first day of the period) reflects if her estrogen levels are normal for her.

Estradiol and FSH are on a similar seesaw as TSH and thyroid hormones or ACTH and cortisol. If estradiol is high for you, then your FSH will be low. If estradiol is low for you, then your FSH will be high. It's very individual.

Let me give you an example: I have twin sisters who have slightly different body types and estrogen levels. Both went through menopause at the same time. The twin with a more athletic build had an estradiol level of 30 which is below normal. The twin with the more curvy figure had an estradiol level of 100 which is normal. Both of their FSHs were very high, well over 80. Both their pituitary glands were screaming at their ovaries to make more estrogen like they did in their youth. Estradiol levels are not always an accurate measurement of a woman's normal ovarian function.

For women who are not cycling due to menopause or I suspect premature ovarian failure, FSH can be drawn anytime. An FSH over 30 is considered menopausal.

In menopausal women, I also draw an lutenizing hormone (LH) to determine how deficient her progesterone is for her. In a reproductive woman, **LH** stimulates ovulation which stimulates ovarian progesterone production.

I only measure progesterone in infertile women to determine if they've ovulated and if they make enough progesterone to carry their baby to term. Progesterone must be drawn seven days before an expected cycle, for example on day 21 in a 28 day cycle.

In a man, LH stimulates testosterone production, while FSH stimulates sperm production. I only draw an FSH if a man's sperm count is low. If I suspect hypogonadism, I draw a LH and testosterone panel to check their hypothalamic-pituitary-testes axis. I look at total **testosterone** and **free testosterone** which is the active form. If free testosterone is low it's usually because sex hormone binding globulin (SHBG) is high.

In both men and women, **SHBG** is created by the liver in response to how much estradiol is synthesized from testosterone. Yes, female ovaries make testosterone first which is then synthesized to estradiol. In postmenopausal women, testosterone is the last hormone to decline usually after age 70.

Dihydrotestosterone (DHT) is the most potent form of testosterone which stimulates muscle mass in men, but also causes male pattern baldness and enlarged prostates. So I include **DHT** in male hormone panels to see how they're converting their native testosterone or testosterone replacement therapy.

A very important hypothalamus hormone that we can measure is prolactin. **Prolactin** has a critical circadian rhythm - high at night and low during the day. I measure prolactin between 8-9 am and expect it to be under 9 ng/ml. And there must be no nipple stimulation at least 24 hours prior to measuring prolactin as nipple stimulation will elevate it.

Then I evaluate human growth hormone (HGH) activity by measuring insulin-like growth factor-1 (IgF-1). **IgF-1** is high in a growing child, stabilizes in young adulthood, and slowly declines at middle age mirroring HGH production over the lifespan.

Last I may run an **ANA** - antinuclear antibody - which is a marker of auto-immunity. If ANA is high then I get specific antibody testing for suspected autoimmune conditions.

In addition I may need other tests to determine hypothalamus dysfunction.

- Blood and urine osmolality - if I suspect issues with vasopressin (ADH)
- Genetic analysis if I suspect Kallman or Prader-Willis
- Visual field test - if I suspect a hypothalamic-pituitary tumor
- Brain MRI - if I suspect a hypothalamic-pituitary tumor

Then according to the patient's history, I order digestive stool analysis. Often to heal the hypothalamus, I have to heal the gut lining first. If I suspect heavy metal exposure, I may order a urine toxicology.

Once I make the diagnosis of hypothalamic dysfunction, treatment varies according to the individual needs of the patient. No two cases are exactly the same. Some patients need full hormone supplementation, others need partial supplementation, most need to make lifestyle modifications and all need nutraceutical hypothalamus support.

What if hypothalamus dysfunction goes untreated?

Well, your symptoms will continue and you will age more rapidly. Plus there's serious complications that will shorten your life.

Hypothalamus hormone deficiencies like low production of TRH or CRH can cause central hypothyroidism and adrenal insufficiency. This may result in heart problems, elevated cholesterol, electrolyte disturbances and low blood pressure. If your GnRH production is low, you can expect weakness, osteoporosis, and high cholesterol. Oxytocin deficiencies and high prolactin can result in infertility, erectile dysfunction, and inorgasmia.

It is vital for your wellbeing and longevity for your hypothalamus to function optimally. Treating lower endocrine gland abnormalities with hormone replacement therapy is a bandaid solution.

One of my patients, a woman in her mid 30's, diagnosed with panhypopituitarism (meaning she made none of her own hormones) and an anatomically normal pituitary gland, came to me wanting bio-identical hormone replacement (BHRT) rather than the synthetics she'd been taking for years. She had never had a period and only with obsessive exercise and complete hormone replacement therapy (estrogen, progesterone, cortisol, DHEA, thyroxine) was she able to keep her weight under control.

She did very well on the BHRT for years. When I finally developed a plant based nutraceutical to support her hypothalamus, she agreed to give it a try. Over the next eighteen months, she was able to wean off all of her hormones, and had her own periods not induced by exogenous hormones. I told her it was time to think about contraception. She laughed. She still believed what the doctors had told her all her life—that she was infertile.

At the age of 43, she gave birth to a healthy baby boy. She has been hormone-free since. I suspect that when she gets close to menopause, she may need some transitional hormone supplementation. If the woman with no hormones can start making her own by optimizing her hypothalamus function, there's hope for all of us.

Addressing the root cause of your health issues means optimizing hypothalamus function.

Thankfully there's a way to support your hypothalamus naturally to optimize its function, keep your Hormones in Harmony®, your immune system protecting you, and your brain working at its best. I'll go into detail in part three.

Hormones over the lifespan

Did you know your hormones are vital over your entire lifespan? Yes, beginning in the womb and through death, your hypothalamus directs your hormones to help you survive.

Most people don't understand that their hormones are part of their physiology, the way their body functions, throughout their life. Hormones are active when you're a fetus even higher than adulthood. Once you're born, your hormones drop down in childhood. You're growing and developing but not as rapidly as you did in the womb.

The first hormone spike happens in puberty when the adrenals start producing more DHEA. Since DHEA can be converted into testosterone and then estrogen, it's adrenal DHEA that initiates signs of puberty - body odor, armpit hair, pubic hair, breast buds.

In girls, the ovaries wake up a year or two after breast buds appear and menstruation begins. Menarchy is the first period. Pubescent boys will start having nocturnal emissions or wet dreams, which is a sign of testicular testosterone production.

Then growth hormone surges. For males it's two to four years after puberty and for females it's approximately 18 months to two years after menarchy. When growth hormone peaks determines final adult height.

Then the basal metabolic rate, which is controlled by the thyroid, rises enough to support all of the growth that's going on during the teen years. Basal metabolic rate or BMR is most rapid in adolescence. In adults, BMR is determined by genetics and more so lifestyle. The more active you are, the higher your BMR. Studies show that your gut microbiome helps to direct your BMR along with your hypothalamus.

In adults, all hormone levels flatten out for two to three decades.

Then very slowly over ten to fifteen years, your hormones decline. We recognize menopause as a distinct hormonal decline. Yet men too go through the change called andropause as their testosterone declines. In fact all of your endocrine glands produce less hormones in the last third of your life.

As they came in, thus they go out. First, the adrenals decline, then the ovaries or testes, then the pituitary, then the thyroid. So many of my patients

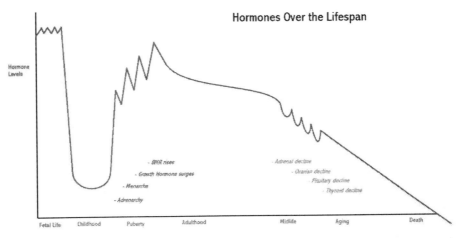

Hormones Over the Lifespan

with hypothyroidism showed signs of adrenal decline and had sex hormone imbalances well before their thyroids became dysfunctional.

When your hormones are low enough, your cells begin to die. Death is the ultimate lack of hormonal communication. Aging gracefully means keeping your hypothalamus functioning optimally so your hormones are in harmony.

Let's meet some hormonally challenged people. They're real patients of mine whose names have been changed. They come in with a multitude of symptoms. They've seen many different healthcare providers. They've tried many different treatments but they're still out of balance. They wish to have their root issue addressed - hypothalamic dysfunction. They are complicated cases with a variety of systems out of balance. The key to their healing is addressing their root issue as well as supporting the systems that are out of balance.

You may recognize yourself.

Part Two

Is this You?

Chapter 4

Infertility, PCOS and Hypothalamic Dysfunction

One beautiful spring morning, Abby comes in to consult with me. At only 27 years old, she already has hormonal issues. Her periods are all over the place - skipping months, then followed by heavy bleeding for weeks. She's overweight with most of her body fat distributed around her middle - an ominous sign of insulin resistance. I suspect she has had polycystic ovary syndrome for years because she was put on a birth control pill to regulate her periods when she was an adolescent.

As a registered nurse, Abby has worked the night shift for over five years. She complains of depression, mostly related to her inability to conceive. She got married a few years ago and has been trying to get pregnant for the past 24 months.

"I just want to have a baby but we can't afford infertility treatments," Abby confides tearfully.

I take her hand. "I'll do my best to help you get pregnant but first, we have to get you healthy."

When I get her on the exam table, I notice that Abby has hirsutism - male like hair growth on her chest, belly, and pubis. Besides carrying the majority of her weight around her middle, she also has some darkening of the skin in her armpits. Acanthosis nigricans are areas of dark, thick velvety skin in body folds and creases, typically affecting the axillae, groin and neck. This type of skin condition is associated with long-term insulin resistance.

An athlete in her teens, Abby is naturally mesomorphic - muscular, not slender. Over the years, she's gained significant weight mostly in her torso. She shows signs of estrogen dominance with heavy breasts which have gotten bigger over the last few years. She also experiences frequent bloating with water retention. Especially around her periods, she can't even wear her rings since her fingers swell like sausages.

On her pelvic exam, Abby's ovaries are normal in size. You don't have to have enlarged ovaries with multiple cysts to have polycystic ovary syndrome. The condition was named when young infertile women with menstrual irregularities were found to have cysts on their ovaries. We now know that these cysts are a natural occurrence when a woman doesn't ovulate regularly. Of course, it's difficult to conceive if you don't ovulate.

What's most concerning to me is Abby's depression. She has had a low mood, poor motivation, difficulty sleeping, and low energy for over a year. She describes herself as a positive person, looking for the best in others and her situation, but her infertility is really affecting her outlook. Her husband is also worried about her and she is worried, too - for herself and her marriage.

Studies show that depression is common in infertility. It makes sense that if you're trying to get pregnant and can't, you might be depressed, but there is a definite neuroendocrine connection. Both your fertility and moods are controlled by your hypothalamus. The hypothalamus directs the production of gonadotropin releasing hormone (GnRH) which stimulates the pituitary gland to produce follicle stimulating hormone (FSH) to initiate the development of ovarian follicles and then luteinizing hormone (LH) to stimulate ovulation.

Your hypothalamus controls your sex hormone production, as well as your neurotransmitter production. Your sex hormones influence your moods.

Estrogen enhances serotonin production which helps modulate your moods and memory. Serotonin disturbances can be influenced by estrogenic status and are at the basis of depression, migraines, irritable bowel syndrome and eating disorders.

Progesterone enhances GABA function, which helps you calm down and sleep. The progesterone metabolite, allopregnanolone, is a GABA receptor agonist binding to GABA receptors and increasing GABA function.

Testosterone influences dopamine production, which enhances your motivation. Dopamine can influence sex steroid production by impacting hypothalamic GnRH. Hormones and neurotransmitters go hand in hand. Keeping your hypothalamus functioning optimally helps balance hormones and neurotransmitters, thus improving your fertility and moods.

PCOS and the hypothalamus

Like all my patients, the first thing I do for Abby is to educate her. I start with explaining the connection between her hypothalamus and her hormone imbalance. Then I teach her how to correct the abnormal hormone metabolism of PCOS.

Polycystic ovary syndrome (PCOS) is a metabolic condition rooted in hypothalamic dysfunction. Eight percent of women of childbearing age are affected by PCOS and commonly present with menstrual irregularities and difficulty conceiving. The androgen excess of PCOS contributes to hirsutism and acne. Women with PCOS are at increased risk for endometrial cancer, type 2 diabetes, hypertension, hyperlipidemia, and cardiovascular disorders. Healing Abby's PCOS is crucial for her fertility, health, and longevity.

Hormonal miscommunication of PCOS begins at the hypothalamic-pituitary-ovarian axis. Hypothalamic GnRH stimulates pituitary FSH and LH production which work in synergy to stimulate follicle development and ovulation.

The ovarian follicle is made up of different layers that produce different sex hormones. The theca cells of the ovarian follicle form an envelope of connective tissue surrounding the granulosa cells. Theca cells are stimulated by LH to produce androgens which then, under the influence of FSH, are converted by aromatase in granulosa cells into estrogens. Insulin influences theca cell hormone production. The theca cells of women with PCOS tend to be insulin resistant.

Circadian rhythms also impact reproduction by controlling many functions in the hypothalamic-pituitary-gonadal axis. By interfering with her day/night cycles, Abby's work has significantly affected her reproduction.

Abnormal activation of hypothalamic GnRH neurons plays a vital role in PCOS development. Hypothalamic GnRH neurons not only control the reproductive axis, but also are the central connection point to metabolic regulation. Metabolic factors such as insulin resistance and obesity in women with PCOS regulate GnRH neuron activity and ultimately reproductive function.

Because women with PCOS do not ovulate regularly, they don't produce enough progesterone. Without enough progesterone, they have a tendency to have too much estrogen activity known as estrogen dominance. Naturally, women make 10 to 50 times more progesterone than estrogen. Progesterone counterbalances estrogen's growth promoting factors.

If estrogen is the fertilizer, progesterone is the gardener.

Estrogen makes everything juicy - cells, skin, mucus membranes. Estrogen stimulates growth of breast cells, the endometrial lining of the uterus, hair, and nails.

Progesterone knows the difference between what should still be growing and what needs to stop growing. When a woman does not get pregnant in a menstrual cycle, progesterone changes the lining of the uterus, allowing it to shed. Progesterone tells breast cells to stop replicating so that tissue doesn't become cancerous. It's vitally important that progesterone and estrogen are in balance. Progesterone turns on the P53 gene which causes cell death in tumor cells.

All hormones have partners. Estrogen's partner is progesterone. Progesterone is also the precursor to cortisol, which helps support adrenal function. Women with PCOS are prone to adrenal issues, particularly high DHEA levels and poor stress response. Lean women with PCOS tend to have higher DHEA levels than obese women with PCOS.

One way to check Abby's potential fertility and diagnose PCOS is to check the anti-Müllerian hormone (AMH) in her blood. AMH is produced by the antral follicles on the ovary when it's getting ready to release an egg. The more antral follicles a woman has, the higher her AMH level will be. Women with PCOS have high AMH levels. If too many follicles try to develop during each menstrual cycle, eggs are wasted. AMH is also a marker of ovarian reserve - meaning the number of eggs that are left. Females are born with 1-2 million primary oocytes but by the time a girl reaches puberty, only about 300,000 eggs have survived. After three decades of menstruating, women run out of eggs and become menopausal. Very low AMH is an indicator of low ovarian reserve. High levels of AMH in PCOS patients often correspond with estrogen dominance.

Estrogen Metabolism

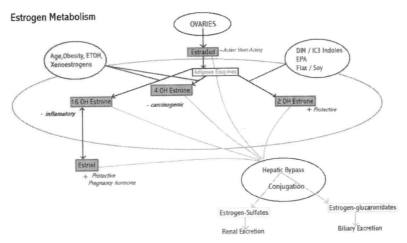

There are three types of estrogen - estradiol, estrone and estriol. While ovarian estradiol is the most potent estrogen, it's very short-acting. Fat cells have an enzyme that converts estradiol into long-acting estrone. All estrogens are 17 carbon molecules, but which carbon has the hydroxyl group determines whether estrone is good, bad or ugly.

2OH-estrone is the good one that is prominently produced in healthy young women, influenced by exercise, dietary IC3 indoles from cruciferous vegetables, fish oils specifically EPA, flax lignans and soy ipriflavones.

4OH-estrone is the bad one, as it's known to be carcinogenic. Conjugated equine estrones derived from pregnant mares' urine and commonly used as oral hormone replacement therapy are predominantly converted into 4OH-estrone.

16OH-estrone is the ugly one - very inflammatory, its conversion is influenced by age, obesity, alcohol overuse and chemical exposures like BPA in plastics, the pesticide DDT, as well as drugs like cimetidine used for ulcers.

Although Abby is young and does not have estrogenic chemical exposures nor abuses alcohol, she does not eat enough fatty fish or cruciferous vegetables, nor does she exercise regularly, and she's overweight. Thankfully, these are lifestyle changes we can help her work on.

I encourage Abby to eat more broccoli, cauliflower, brussel sprouts, and kale so she has more IC_3 indoles, specifically more diindolymethane (DIM), available for safer estradiol conversion. Three to four servings of fatty fish a week will help, as well as adding flax into her diet. I am careful about encouraging too much soy intake as excess soy can interfere with T_3 activity. So, I advise her to limit soy protein to less than 20 gm per day.

I also recommend that Abby start exercising. Although she's always on her feet at night as a nurse, she tends to be sedentary at home. Studies show that getting up every half hour and walking around for five minutes can help reduce the effects of being sedentary. So, we start by encouraging Abby to get moving, before working on more formal exercise activities. I've found that encouraging my patients to take baby steps in changing their lifestyle is much more likely to become their permanent habits. It takes at least 40 days to create a habit. So, to help set my patients up for success, our therapeutic plans are in six week intervals.

Thankfully, excess 16OH-estrone can be converted into protective estriol. Estriol is the dominant estrogen of pregnancy, encourages healthy skin, hair and mucus membranes, but is not potent enough for neuroprotection, which is why I prefer estradiol as hormone replacement therapy.

We can run urine or blood tests to determine Abby's estrogen conversion - specifically her ratio of 16OH to 2OH estrone - and then recommend intense supplementation like DIM and flax lignans to improve her conversion. Since most women with PCOS have elevated 16OH to 2OH estrone ratios, we start with nutritional and lifestyle changes.

When no longer needed by the body, all hormones, including estrogens, go through the liver for detoxification. Liver enzymes make cholesterol dominant hormones water soluble. Then the liver handcuffs steroid hormones in a process called conjugation before releasing them into the bile to be dumped into the intestine. Sulfated estrogen is returned to the bloodstream to be urinated out of the body. Gluconated estrogens are defecated out of the body.

All of your hormones go through this detoxification process and are conjugated with different peptides - adrenal and thyroid hormones, insulin, growth hormone - all hormones. That's why liver health is so important. For this young woman with signs of estrogen dominance, we also focus on her liver and gut health. Why her gut? Because if she has an unhealthy gut microbiome, she will recycle her estrogens increasing her estrogen dominance. Healthy balanced gut flora helps detox and metabolize hormones. We can test her gut hormone metabolism by collecting stool and measuring beta-glucuronidase - an enzyme produced by the gut microbiome that in excess will break the handcuffs on detoxified estrogens, which will then be reabsorbed by the intestine. If Abby has high beta-glucuronidase in her stool, we can give her calcium-d-glucarate to block the effects of the enzyme until we get her gut flora back in balance.

Balancing hormones means assessing all the body's systems, including digestion and detoxification.

PCOS and Insulin Resistance

In PCOS, I want to correct insulin resistance. While I will recommend an insulin resistant diet, I need to check Abby's blood glucose levels. So, I'm going to include in her blood work - hemoglobin A1C. As suspected, Abby's HGBA1C is elevated at 5.9%.

Hemoglobin A1C (HGBA1C) is a peptide on the red blood cells. If your blood glucose runs high, HGBA1C will be elevated. HGBA1C over 5.6%

indicates insulin resistance, over 6.1% indicates diabetes. While fasting blood glucose levels are important, HGBA1C gives us a better baseline as it reflects average blood sugars over the past six to eight weeks, which is the lifespan of a red blood cell.

To check the amount of insulin Abby's pancreas is making, I order a C-peptide. Pancreatic beta cells produce pro-insulin which separates into insulin and C-peptide. C-peptide has a longer circulating half-life of 30 minutes compared to the 5 to 10 minute half-life of insulin making it a useful measurement of insulin production. C-peptide is elevated in patients with insulin resistance, early type 2 diabetes, obesity and glucose intolerance. C-peptide is decreased in patients with type 1 diabetes and long standing type 2 diabetes when the worn out pancreas can no longer produce enough insulin. Abby's c-peptide is elevated, indicating her insulin levels are high which is common with insulin resistance.

Next, I teach Abby how her hormones get into her cells. Since she has signs of insulin resistance, I focus on the insulin receptor.

All hormones, neurotransmitters, and immune cytokines need receptor sites to affect cell function. Some of these messengers - like sex steroids and thyroid hormones - enter the cell membrane through the receptor sites. Some like serotonin and dopamine only need to dock into the receptor site to activate cell function. Insulin has an interesting relationship with cell receptor sites.

Cell membranes are composed of glycoproteins surrounding phospholipids. Think of the cell membrane as a butter sandwich with the bread being the glycoprotein layers and the butter being the phospholipid layer. In the butter sandwich are pitted olives. They represent doorways into the cells - receptor sites.

Effective receptor sites require healthy cell membranes. Cell membranes become thin and ineffective with age, malnutrition, disease and toxicity. Think of receptor sites as locks and hormones, neurotransmitters and cytokines as keys. Every biochemical messenger key has its own very specific receptor site lock. While not all biochemical messengers have receptor sites on every cell, all cells do have insulin receptors. Since glucose is vital for cell energy production, cell membranes must have insulin receptors to function.

Insulin resistance is a cell membrane issue. When cells are over exposed to glucose and insulin, they can develop resistance. This means that not all of their insulin receptor sites function. This is a protective measure for cells that cannot store glucose. Your heart cells, for instance, can only use glucose for energy to pump or to grow. Once your heart reaches its adult size, it cannot grow any larger and be an effective pump. If you have too much insulin and sugar floating around, your heart cells become resistant to insulin to prevent abnormal growth. You can store the extra glucose in your liver and muscles as glycogen - but only 400 calories worth. The rest gets packaged by your liver into triglycerides for storage in your fat cells. That's why we refer to the extra fat around your middle as your insulin meter. The thicker the belly fat in your insulin meter, the higher your insulin has been and the more insulin resistant you are.

Effects of Insulin

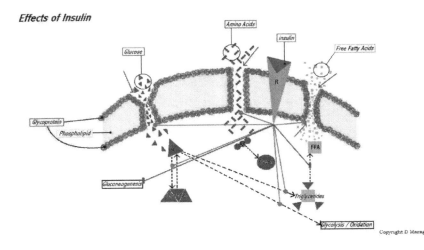

Copyright D Maragopoulos 2016

Insulin escorts glucose to your cells. When insulin docks on its receptor site, the cell membrane opens up gateways to allow glucose to enter the cell. Glucose then enters the cell mitochondria to be converted into adenosine triphosphate (ATP) energy. Insulin also unlocks gateways for amino acids, fatty acids and water to move in and out of the cells. When a person is insulin resistant, they're not just missing their glucose and producing less energy, instead they're missing amino acids and fatty acids. Amino acids are the building blocks, not just to build muscle, bone, and tissues but also to build enzymes, hormones, neurotransmitters and cytokines. Free fatty acids are part of tissue building blocks, too. Without the free flow of water in and out of the membrane, cells become dehydrated and toxic from their own waste.

Insulin resistant cells cannot function properly. Thyroid cells can't make as much thyroid hormone. Liver cells don't produce enough bile. Insulin resistant cells cannot repair themselves, detoxify properly and are dehydrated. Insulin resistance affects everything. So, it's so important that insulin resistance is addressed.

Treating insulin resistance is key to resolving PCOS

Since Abby's HBGA1C is elevated, we will initiate lifestyle measures like an insulin resistant diet and exercise plus add berberine to help reverse her insulin resistance. Berberine has been shown to work similarly to metformin, a diabetic drug used for PCOS.

A bio active botanical, berberine, is a yellow-colored alkaloid that is used to treat diabetes, hypercholesterolemia, inflammation, obesity, and PCOS. Like metformin, berberine affects adenosine monophosphate kinase (AMPK), the enzyme that controls cell energy production. Berberine has the same effect on insulin resistance and fat loss as increasing exercise while restricting calorie intake.

Berberine has been shown to increase glycolysis - breaking down glucose inside cells - decrease glucose production in the liver, and slow the breakdown of carbohydrates in the gut. Berberine can also help restore the microbiome of the gut, which has been shown to help increase body fat loss.

Studies in diabetics show that one gram of berberine per day can lower fasting blood sugar by 20% and lower HGBA1C by 12%. In head-to-head studies, berberine was better than metformin in reducing waist size and waist-to-hip ratio.

In studies on women with PCOS, berberine effectively blocked glucose uptake and excessive testosterone production of insulin-resistant theca cells. Berberine can help reduce acne and lower testosterone levels that contribute to hirsutism. Berberine also helps to improve fertility in women with PCOS.

Although berberine is an effective alternative to metformin, it is important to note that it is not meant for long-term use.

This is why I focus on supporting the hypothalamus. The hypothalamus controls glucose metabolism, blood pressure, inflammation, hormones, and fertility. If the hypothalamus is supported nutraceutically, then three months of berberine use is usually sufficient to correct insulin resistance.

Completing the infertility evaluation

As part of Abby's infertility work up, I order a semen analysis for her husband. I want to be sure he has enough normal mobile healthy sperm before putting her through more invasive testing. If she had chlamydia when she was younger or an ovarian cyst that ruptured and caused some adhesions, I will need to determine the patency of her fallopian tubes.

A hysterosalpingogram is an imaging study where dye is inserted through the cervix, moves up through the uterus and hopefully through the fallopian tubes. If there are light adhesions in the fallopian tube, sometimes a hysterosalpingogram can clear the blockage. Since fertilization usually occurs in the fallopian tubes, a hysterosalpingogram will reveal if the path the sperm must take to meet the ovum is clear or not.

If we determine by her luteal phase progesterone level that Abby is ovulating yet she still is not conceiving, then we will want to be sure her cervical mucus is not hostile. The spermatozoa must utilize the cervical mucus to access the uterus. Sometimes a man's sperm is not compatible with a woman's cervical mucus. She produces antibodies and the sperm dies before entering her uterus. So, we do a postcoital test.

I will ask the couple to abstain from intercourse for two days before ovulation, and then have intercourse 2-8 hours prior to the office visit for the postcoital test. They should not use a lubricant during sex and definitely no douching or submerging in water after sex, but taking a shower is permissible. During a pelvic exam, I will take two samples - one from the vaginal cul de sac beneath the cervix and one from the endocervical canal. Then I compare the samples under the microscope looking for live spermatozoa. If the sperm is mobile in the vaginal sample but not in the endocervical sample, then the cervical mucus is considered hostile. If so, Abby will need intrauterine insemination to bypass her cervical mucus and give her husband's sperm a fighting chance to fertilize an ovum. Many gynecological practices bypass this simple but necessary part of the evaluation – oftentimes, for lack of a microscope in the office.

Cervical incompetence is more prevalent in pregnant women with PCOS so once Abby gets pregnant we will be monitoring her pregnancy closely. Cervical incompetence means the cervix does not stay closed and can result in second trimester miscarriage and prematurity. Other factors contributing to cervical incompetence include cervical procedures like LEEP, cryotherapy, or cold knife conization. Fortunately, Abby has never had an abnormal Pap smear so has never needed a cervical procedure.

Getting pregnant naturally

Abby's number one goal is to get pregnant. While I will focus on restoring her fertility, I make sure she understands that restoring her health and specifically optimizing her hypothalamus function will better insure having a healthy baby. We begin by supporting her hypothalamus nutraceutically with Genesis Gold®. Since Genesis Gold® has been available, I do much less classic infertility treatments or refer patients for IVF.

Why? Because optimizing hypothalamus function helps restore fertility by improving sex steroid production, reducing insulin resistance, improving immune and other endocrine function that may inhibit reproduction. Your hypothalamus' job is to be sure you're healthy enough to conceive, otherwise you're passing on your health issues to your child.

We make sure that Abby is eating a super clean diet and avoiding environmental toxins. We want her as healthy as possible before conceiving. Her potential embryos' genetics are stored in her gametes. Three months before conceiving, a woman's gametes' DNA is vulnerable to environmental influences; a man's spermatozoa are susceptible eight weeks before conception. So, both partners must clean up their acts to help insure a healthy baby. Their future child will also benefit from their father optimizing his hypothalamus function.

In terms of other lab testing besides HGBA1C and c-peptide, I check Abby's adrenal and thyroid function as well as prolactin levels. As expected, her androgens both DHEA-S and testosterone are elevated.

Her full thyroid panel including TSH, fT4, fT3 are within normal limits and communicating well with each other, which is important because hypothyroidism can interfere with fertility. Keeping a pregnant woman's TSH about 2.5mIU/L helps ensure healthy fetal brain development.

High prolactin can interfere with fertility and needs to be addressed sooner than later. Thankfully, Abby's 8 am prolactin is within normal circadian rhythm.

I also run a full chemistry panel to make sure her liver and kidneys are healthy, with a CBC to be sure she's not anemic. Some women with PCOS bleed heavily when they do have periods. Abby's chemistry and CBC are normal.

We check Abby's progesterone level in her luteal phase to determine if she is ovulating and making enough progesterone to maintain the pregnancy for the first fourteen weeks until the placenta is mature enough to produce progesterone.

The little cave left over after a mature follicle ovulates is called the corpus luteum. The corpus luteum becomes an active endocrine gland producing progesterone to stabilize the lining of the uterus. The high levels of estrogen produced in the follicular phase of the menstrual cycle build up the endometrial lining, but it's progesterone that makes the endometrial lining involute to allow implantation to occur. Without adequate levels of progesterone, a fertilized ovum would be shed prematurely. A woman who ovulates but does not make enough progesterone to maintain a pregnancy has a corpus luteal defect.

Thankfully, Abby notices spinbarkheidt - a slick elongated mucus produced by the cervix at ovulation under the influence of high estrogen levels. Spinbarkheidt enables the spermatozoa to enter the cervical os (opening).

Since Abby's periods are irregular, we need to use her cervical mucus to help determine the proper time to check her progesterone. Once she notices spinbarkheidt, I ask her to use an over the counter fertility urine test that detects LH. Seven to nine days after her LH surge, we check her serum progesterone.

Abby's results show that she is ovulating but does not make enough progesterone to sustain a pregnancy. Like most of my PCOS patients, Abby will need extra progesterone in the first trimester of pregnancy to prevent early miscarriage.

My assessment of Abby is hypothalamus dysfunction with polycystic ovary condition, insulin resistance, infertility and depression.

Since Abby has been metabolically out of balance since her teens, we will need to support optimal hypothalamus function for at least ten months, although I expect regulation of her menstrual cycles, sensitization of her insulin receptors and balancing of her neurotransmitters within the first two to three months, and conception within six to twelve months.

Here's what Abby's healing plan looks like:

1. Hypothalamic support - I recommended Genesis Gold® 4gm of powder mixed in water per fifty pounds of body weight taken every morning at least fifteen minutes before eating breakfast. My PCOS patients often become pregnant within 3-6 months of taking Genesis Gold® without any other intervention. I expect her periods to regulate within this amount of time.

2. Nutrition - Before initiating an insulin resistant diet, I recommend a liver cleanse diet. Not because I suspect Abby has liver disease or is particularly toxic, but because she does not have the best dietary habits. It will be easier for her to stick with the low carb insulin resistant diet after cleaning out her liver for three days by eating lots of vegetables but no fat or protein. I calculate her current lean body mass to be 100 pounds and recommend at least 50 gm of protein and 25 gm of fat daily once she starts the insulin resistant diet. Her dietary focus is health, reduction of insulin resistance and loss of body fat.

3. Activity - Abby will have to adopt a more active lifestyle. We focus on getting her to start by power walking for ten minutes three times a day. We will have her work up to 20-30 minutes of aerobic activity 3-5 times per week. I want her to be successful, so baby steps.

4. Sleep - Since Abby works 12 hour night shifts three days per week, we are going to optimize her melatonin production by making sure her room is completely dark and she doesn't eat within three hours of going to sleep. We want her to get at least 20 minutes of daylight exposure so she has to get up before dusk. That will be her best time to exercise, too. On her days off, we will encourage her to sleep at night if possible.

5. Mindset - While Abby is highly motivated, she's been dealing with her health issues for a while and is feeling depressed. Helping her adopt a more healing mindset means helping her work though her situational and hormonally triggered depression. I recommend meditation, journaling her feelings, keeping a dream journal as I expect her sleep to deepen and her dreams to become more lucid with hypothalamus support. Oftentimes in your dreams, subconscious limiting beliefs can make themselves known. I will recommend therapy if she is unable to commit to some of the self-reflection techniques. I will also recommend joining a support group, in person or virtually as her time is limited. Finding a circle of supportive people can be instrumental to staying accountable to her healing goals.

6. For intense treatment of insulin resistance and the androgenic aspects of PCOS - I recommend Berberine 500 mg with at least two meals per day. I advise her to introduce Berberine slowly, starting with her biggest meal which should be lunch for a few days before adding it to a second meal. Berberine is high in tannins, which can cause gastric upset. I advise her to report any side effects like rash or headache.

7. To treat corpus luteal defect - I recommend transdermal progesterone in a liposomal base 50 mg twice daily from ovulation through the first fourteen weeks of pregnancy. If she starts bleeding about the time of an expected menstruation, she is not to stop the progesterone until she confirms she is not pregnant with a urine test. Any early pregnancy bleeding indicates she may need more progesterone. She has a standing order for a serum HCG to confirm pregnancy and serum progesterone level to be sure she's taking enough.

Results

After consulting with me, Abby decides to wait a few months to get herself as healthy as possible to conceive. Abby joins our Hormone Healing Circle for compassionate support and accountability to help her stick with her new lifestyle changes. She discovers through the virtual group experience that as much as she desires to have children, she is concerned about becoming a mother, needs better communication with her spouse, and desperately wants to be at her optimal state of health and well-being before getting pregnant. It's a delight to be part of this young woman's healing journey.

By the end of the first month of hypothalamic support, Abby notices a significant change in her mood. She becomes hopeful and is no longer feeling depressed and is sleeping much more deeply. Within three months of hypothalamic support, diet, exercise, and berberine, Abby loses her extra body fat, her HGBA1C drops down to 5.5%, her c-peptide drops as well, indicating her pancreas is no longer having to make high levels of insulin. Her periods have become regular and she feels ready to try and conceive. She stops taking berberine but continues phase two of the insulin resistant diet and her new exercise regimen.

By the fifth month, Abby is pregnant with her first child. She uses transdermal progesterone as prescribed until her second trimester. She chooses to continue to take Genesis Gold® and has a lovely uneventful pregnancy – thankfully, no gestational diabetes nor pregnancy induced hypertension which is common in PCOS. She delivers a healthy baby girl near term with no postpartum depression and successfully nurses her daughter for over a year. Abby is happy with her health and hormonal balance and plans to continue to support her hypothalamus throughout her reproductive years.

Chapter 5

Hypothyroidism, Virility and Your Hypothalamus

At 38 years old, Doug is pretty seriously distressed over his low testosterone. He's been losing his hair for a few years with classic male pattern baldness at the temples. Doug is a fireman on the force for 15 years and complains that he has not been able to keep up with his fitness program because his energy is low. Doug's gained weight and is disgusted with what he calls his "man boobs".

He also noticed he's lost his confidence. A divorcée, Doug's low libido and issues with sexual performance prevents him from participating in the dating world. Doug is a father of three children, ages 5, 8 and 11 and has been struggling sharing custody with his alcoholic ex-wife.

Doug was diagnosed a few years earlier with Hashimoto's thyroiditis and started taking synthetic thyroid hormone. While increasing his energy for the first six months, levothyroxine seemed to stop working and his energy plummeted about a year later. That's when he noticed the weight gain, hair loss, and being cold all the time.

"My doctor keeps telling me that my bloodwork is fine. But I don't feel fine." Doug shakes his head. "I'm sick and tired of the run around. There must be something that can be done."

I nod, "There is. We need to figure out what's at the root of your health issues."

Being a fireman, Doug has been exposed to inhalant chemicals, long work hours, crazy sleep schedules, and lots of stress. He's on his own now without a significant other, juggling childcare and worries when his wife has the children. He admits to living in co-dependent relationships from childhood with a bipolar mother. Doug has a lot of work to do and I'm here to help him get started on his healing journey.

Doug's history is typical of many stressed individuals whose work has disrupted their normal circadian rhythm. He says he has trouble sleeping, so he doesn't go to sleep when he should, and is suffering from sleep deprivation.

When he does get up in the morning, it takes him hours before he feels like he's not sleepwalking. He uses caffeine to try to wake up and will go through a half a pot of coffee without much change in his energy. Doug reports that he tries to keep moving because if he sits still, he's likely to doze off. That is typical of hypothyroidism.

His diet log reveals that he's consuming too much sugar in the form of energy drinks and too much fat with not nearly enough vegetables.

Doug says he's too busy to do any type of meditation and his spiritual practice is limited to bedtime prayers with his children.

Like most of my patients, Doug brings in his latest labs. His thyroid antibodies are still elevated in spite of being on levothyroxine for years. His T_3 levels are low and his TSH is severely suppressed with low normal T_4. That's a sure sign of hypothalamic-pituitary-thyroid (HPT) axis dysfunction, which is not uncommon when you put patients on high levels of synthetic thyroid hormone.

His sex steroids are also affected with low testosterone, high dihydrotestos-terone (DHT) and elevated estradiol. Doug says he's tried maca, a herb that has androgenic properties, but it didn't help much.

I note that the back of Doug's upper arm muscles are flat - a sign of testoster-one deficiency. The deltoid is a large muscle made of three parts attaching the arm to the shoulder. The back or posterior deltoid is testosterone depen-dent. Women have to be incredible athletes doing a lot of shoulder work to develop the posterior deltoid. In adolescence, men's posterior deltoids develop naturally at puberty and start to flatten out when their testosterone levels fall at midlife. Except Doug is only 38.

In the past 25 years, I've noticed that even young men have much less poste-rior deltoid development and more midline body fat than ever before. That suggests testosterone levels are falling and conversion to estrogen is rising. Doug's high DHT is causing his male pattern baldness. We can follow Doug's active testosterone by checking his sex hormone binding globulin (SHBG), which if elevated will lower his free testosterone levels.

On his physical exam, I assess that Doug's heart is strong and his lungs are clear. Other than alopecia (hair loss), his head and neck is within normal limits except his thyroid is enlarged. The thyroid is a butterfly-shaped gland that lies around the trachea. It's easiest to feel when you place your fingers around the trachea and have the patient swallow which moves the lobes of the thyroid up against your fingertips to check for size and modularity. If the thyroid is grossly enlarged, it can sometimes feel like you have a lump at the base of your throat when you're swallowing or even talking. A goiter is a gross enlargement of the thyroid, usually seen in autoimmune hypothyroid-ism. Goiters are more common in people who live far inland and do not have access to seafood, which may lead to iodine deficiency.

On breast exam - yes, I examine the male chest for mammary glandular tis-sue, nipple discharge, and adenopathy enlarged lymph nodes - I note that Doug does not have developed mammary glands or nipple discharge but he does have large fat depots under his areolas.

Before adjusting his thyroid hormones and prescribing testosterone, I get a fuller blood panel including a morning prolactin.

Here are Doug's significant lab findings:

- Prolactin high at 67 ng/ml
- Testosterone low normal at 348 ng/dl with low LH at 2IU/l which indicates hypothalamus-pituitary-gonadal (HPG) axis issues, high normal DHT at 90 ng/dl probably contributing to his alopecia
- TSH low at 0.5mIU/l, fT4 low end of normal at 0.8ng/dl, fT3 low end of normal at 2.3 pg/ml, which indicates suppresses HPT axis and TPOab grossly elevated at 600 IU/ml
- LDL cholesterol elevated at 130 mg/dl with small particle pattern B indicating he's eating too many carbs and not getting enough exer-cise which will increase his risk arteriosclerosis
- HGBA1C elevated at 5.9% which indicates insulin resistance

As suspected, Doug has elevated prolactin. An MRI rules out a pituitary tumor. His prolactin is high enough to suppress his receptor sites. With high prolactin, Doug will not feel the benefits of testosterone or a change in thy-roid medication. So first thing first, we have to get his prolactin lowered in the daytime so he has more energy and then prolactin will naturally rise at night and help him sleep.

Prolactin - the Forgotten Hormone

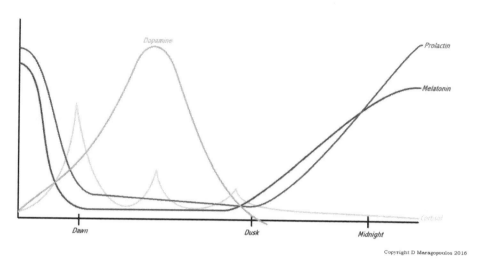

Copyright D Maragopoulos 2016

Prolactin is one of the most underappreciated hormones. I rarely see clinicians checking prolactin levels unless they suspect a patient has a pituitary tumor. It's a shame because high daytime prolactin can be at the root of so many issues.

Prolactin was named for its first recognized function to promote lactation, but it does so much more. Prolactin (PRL) has over 300 functions in the human body, which are classified in six main categories: 1) water and electrolyte equilibrium, 2) growth and development, 3) endocrinology and metabolism, 4) brain and behavior, 5) reproduction and maintaining pregnancy, and 6) immunoregulation and protection.

Prolactin is produced by the hypothalamus and stored in the pituitary gland. Under the influence of hypothalamic prolactin releasing hormone (PRH), the pituitary gland releases prolactin. Prolactin is a nocturnal hormone - meaning that it's produced at highest levels at night and lowest during the day. To determine proper circadian rhythm, I check prolactin between 8-9:00 am in the morning.

Prolactin follows melatonin production by about three hours. Melatonin levels rise about three hours after dusk and peak from 2-4:00 am. Prolactin begins rising around midnight, peaking about 4-7:00 am.

A few hours after dawn, prolactin drops to its low daytime levels. What turns prolactin off is hypothalamic dopamine production. Dopamine is considered prolactin inhibiting hormone (PIH).

Men tend to have lower prolactin levels of about 2-20 ng/dl compared to women at 3-30 ng/dl. Prolactin rises at night to over high teens in men and over twenty in females. If you have normal dopamine production in the morning, then prolactin should be around 9 ng/dl by 9am.

Elevated morning prolactin indicates poor sleep, not getting up with the sun, nipple stimulation within 24 hours of drawing prolactin, autoimmunity, obesity, hypothalamic dopamine deficiency and sometimes a prolactin secreting tumor.

You definitely do not want your prolactin high during the day. Why?

At night, prolactin is released to help your immune system do its job better. It tells your thymus to program WBCs properly and then release them as T-cells. T-cells attack invading microbes and cancer cells.

If prolactin is high during the day, your immune system does not function properly. T-cells attack normal tissue, which is known as autoimmunity. You may not have classic autoimmunity like rheumatoid arthritis, lupus or thyroiditis, but you have autoimmune tendencies. You get rashes easily. You may have leaky gut syndrome. You will have trouble losing weight. The majority of my morbidly obese patients have dyscircadian prolactin levels.

Prolactin causes inhibition of gonadotropin-releasing hormone (GnRH) leading to inhibition of luteinizing hormone (LH) and follicle-stimulating hormone (FSH) secretion. Symptoms of hypogonadism (poor gonad function and low sex steroid production) depend upon the magnitude of prolactin elevation.

Women with serum prolactin greater than 100 ng/dl will have overt hypogonadism which looks like menopausal symptoms - amenorrhea, hot flashes, and vaginal dryness. Serum prolactin between 50 to 100 ng/dl may cause oligomenorrhea (infrequent periods). Serum prolactin between 20 to 50 ng/dl may shorten the luteal phase because of insufficient progesterone secretion which can cause difficulty conceiving and maintaining pregnancy resulting in miscarriage.

In men, serum prolactin greater than 50 ng/dl causes hypogonadotropic hypogonadism, leading to low testosterone production, low libido, impotency, infertility, oligospermia, gynecomastia (breast tissue development), rarely galactorrhea (milk production production), loss of muscle mass, increase body fat and low bone mass.

When hyperprolactinemia is suspected, these labs should be checked to be sure hypothalamic-pituitary function is not affected; serum prolactin, thyroid function test (TSH, fT_4, fT_3), renal function test (BUN, creatinine), insulin-like growth factor-1 (IGF-1), adrenocorticotrophic hormone (ACTH), luteinizing hormone (LH), follicle-stimulating hormone (FSH), testosterone or estradiol.

At 67 ng/dl, Doug's prolactin is way too high, not just dyscircadian.

While I didn't suspect a tumor as he did not have classic symptoms of headache, visual disturbance and milky nipple discharge, I ordered an MRI to be sure. A large enough tumor of the pituitary gland causes significant pressure on the optic nerve. The pituitary sits in a small body space called the sella tursica or Turkish saddle. If your pituitary is any bigger than it's supposed to be, it presses on that bone and causes headaches. Peripheral vision is also disturbed as the enlarged pituitary pushes on the optic nerves.

A prolactin producing tumor or prolactinoma may also induce milky breast discharge both in women and men. Breastfeeding women are supposed to have high levels of prolactin. Prolactin is also elevated in pregnancy to help maintain the pregnancy and protect the mother from the high growth promoting pregnancy hormones by blocking her hormone receptor sites. But if you're not pregnant and prolactin is high during the day, it will eventually block hormone receptors and effectively make you feel like your hormones are too low.

Many of my patients come to me feeling hormonally deficient but have been told by their doctors that their hormone levels are normal. Except they didn't measure prolactin. If prolactin is way above circadian levels, then it's blocking the hormones' ability to get into the cells. So, we must focus on getting prolactin down during the day.

Naturally, at dawn, blue light waves inhibit further melatonin production. Melatonin drops with the sunrise. Your hypothalamus switches to daytime mode, but your glucose is low because, of course, you've been fasting and not eating all night long. So, your hypothalamus stimulates your adrenals to release cortisol. Cortisol stimulates pancreatic glucagon production which releases sugar stored in your liver into your bloodstream. When your hypothalamus uptakes morning glucose, it produces a surge of dopamine. Dopamine shuts prolactin down, wakes you up and your day begins.

Nocturnal prolactin is up for about eight hours. So, if you are going to bed really late, say two o'clock in the morning, and you have to get up at eight, you still have prolactin on board until 10 o'clock in the morning. So, it's like you're sleepwalking. You'll need a lot of caffeine to do anything in the morning.

The most effective way to lower prolactin and reset circadian rhythm is using a short acting dopamine agonist. I prefer bromocryptine tablets as they can be used vaginally or rectally to avoid side effects of oral usage. When taken orally, dopamine agonists can increase blood pressure and cause headaches. Studies show that bypassing the liver using mucus membranes like the vagina or rectum decreases side effects.

I always prescribe bromocryptine to be inserted by 8am after urination or a bowel movement to prevent losing the medication. The tablets usually dissolve within 15-30 minutes and are very effective. Unless a patient has a prolactin secreting tumor that we are trying to shrink, I do not prescribe dopamine agonists to be used around the clock as I do not want to suppress nocturnal prolactin.

Besides hyperprolactinemia, Doug also has hypothyroiditis.

Your Thyroid affects your Basal Metabolic Rate

Thyroid conditions are fairly easy to diagnose. We can see from your TSH if your thyroid is producing enough thyroid hormone, but just measuring TSH is not enough.

What we need to know is if your hypothalamic-pituitary-thyroid axis is functioning properly. So, along with TSH, we need to measure the free active thyroid hormones tetraiodothyronine (fT_4) and triiodothyronine (fT_3).

Regulation of thyroid hormone starts in the hypothalamus. The hypothalamus releases thyrotropin-releasing hormone (TRH) into the hypothalamic-hypophyseal portal system to the anterior pituitary gland. TRH stimulates thyrotropin cells in the anterior pituitary to release TSH.

Released into the bloodstream, TSH binds to the thyroid-releasing hormone receptor (TSH-R) on the basolateral aspect of the thyroid follicular cell. Under the influence of TSH, thyrocytes in the thyroid follicles produce a protein called thyroglobulin (TG).

The thyroid then iodinates thyroglobulin to create thyroid hormones. Iodine is important for thyroid function. T_4 has four iodine molecules and T_3 has only three iodine molecules.

Thyroid peroxidase is an enzyme produced by the thyroid that directs the iodination of thyroglobulin into thyroid hormones. Thyroid peroxidase antibodies are grossly elevated in autoimmune thyroiditis, which usually results in low thyroid function or hypothyroiditis.

Autoimmune thyroiditis or Hashimoto's thyroiditis is named after Dr. Hashimoto, who discovered thyroid auto-antibodies which interfere with normal thyroid function.

In autoimmune hyperthroiditis or Grave's disease, TSH is suppressed by elevated antibodies known as thyroid-stimulating immunoglobulin (TSI). Thyrotropin receptor antibody (TRAb) overrides the normal hypothalamus regulation of the thyroid, causing an overproduction of thyroid hormones (hyperthyroidism).

Thyroid hormones are lipophilic and bind to transport proteins. Only a fraction (approximately 0.2%) of the thyroid hormone is unbound and active. Thyroxine-binding globulin (TBG) transports two-thirds of T_4. When it reaches its target site, T_3 and T_4 can dissociate from their binding protein to enter cells.

While thyroid receptors can bind to both T_3 and T_4, they have a much higher affinity for T_3. As a result, T_4 is relatively inactive, so T_4 must be deiodinated into T_3. If the wrong iodine molecule is removed, it's called reverse T_3 (rT_3) and doesn't fit in the cell receptor site. T_3 must get into your cells and stimulate the mitochondria to produce ATP energy. Energy production raises body heat called thermogenesis. That's why basal body temperature (BBT) is a useful diagnostic tool for assessing thyroid hormone activity.

Thyroid hormone affects virtually every organ system in the body, including the heart, central nervous system, autonomic nervous system, bone, gastro-intestinal system, and cellular metabolism. Essentially, thyroid hormone directs your basal metabolic rate - or how much energy you need to produce to survive.

The hypothalamic-pituitary-thyroid axis is the best example we can see in your blood of the negative feedback system.

If your T_4 and T_3 levels are low, TSH will be high. If T_4 and T_3 levels are high, TSH will be low. Remember it's the hypothalamus that responds to T_4 and T_3 levels to make TRH to stimulate the pituitary to make TSH.

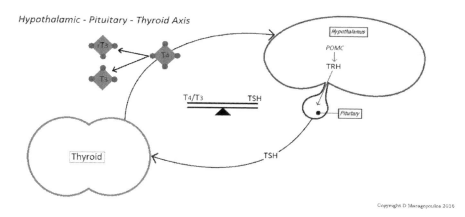

Copyright D. Maragopoulos 2016

If TSH is not responding to T_4/T_3 levels appropriately, that indicates that the hypothalamic-pituitary-thyroid (HPT) axis is dysfunctional. If TSH is high normal with high normal T_4/T_3 that's a dysfunctional HPT axis. If TSH is low with low normal T_4/T_3 as in Doug's case, that's also a dysfunctional HPT axis. If the HPT axis is functional, TSH should be low if thyroid hormones are high or high if thyroid hormones are low.

Besides the negative feedback system, growth hormone, cortisol, and dopamine inhibit TSH production. Cold, stress, and exercise increase TSH production by increasing hypothalamic TRH release.

In autoimmune thyroiditis, the immune system produces antibodies that work against the production of thyroid hormone. Anti-TPO antibody blocks the TPO enzyme which prevents the iodination of thyroid hormones. Anti-TGB antibody binds thyroglobulin preventing adequate thyroid hormone production.

Doug has Hashimoto's thyroiditis with very high anti-TPO antibodies and his high dose synthetic levothyroxin is suppressing his TSH with inadequate levels of T_4 and T_3.

Conventional medicine does not take this functional approach to hypothyroiditis . The belief is that if you give a patient enough synthetic levothyroxine to suppress his TSH, the auto-antibodies will go down. As in most of the patients I consult with, that wasn't the case with Doug.

Auto-thyroid antibodies will not come down unless we support the hypothalamus. Over the past twenty years, I've found that supporting the hypothalamus with Genesis Gold® and extra Sacred Seven® hypothalamic amino acids will result in lowered auto-antibodies. That's because the hypothalamus controls the immune system and unless it's supported, the autoimmune attack continues. We need to stop the autoimmune attack to allow the thyroid to make its own hormones. Right now, Doug is dependent on thyroid replacement therapy.

When I first prescribe thyroid hormone, I usually recommend taking it just six days a week. Taking a break helps to reestablish hypothalamic-pituitary-thyroid communication. Over time with hypothalamic support, we can lower exogenous thyroid hormone dependency as endogenous production kicks in. If you take a hormone your body should be making, that gland may lose its ability to make the hormone which is why most people with hypothyroidism take thyroid hormone for the rest of their lives.

Basal body temperature is one of the best ways to evaluate thyroid hormone activity, particularly if T_3 is getting into the cells and raising the metabolism. Cellular metabolic activity involves the production of energy and heat - thermogenesis.

So, I ask Doug to record his basal body temperature (BBT). I prefer oral temperatures to axillary as hormonally challenged people often have very different skin and core temperatures. He takes his temperature first thing in the morning before getting out of bed for at least three mornings. Normal BBT should be between 97.8 to 98.2 degrees Fahrenheit. As suspected, Doug's BBT is low, averaging 97.2, which means his T_3 activity is low. We will use his BBT to help determine changes in his basal metabolic rate.

Based on his low BBT, low free T_3, low free T_4 and suppressed TSH, I switch Doug to a glandular form of thyroid replacement therapy until he can make enough of his own T_3.

Desiccated thyroid extract is the oldest form of thyroid hormone replacement originally derived from cows in the early 1900s. The T_4 to T_3 ratio is always the same: $38mcgT_4:9mcgT_3$ per grain of desiccated thyroid. I've found that when patients come to me on long-term synthetic thyroid replacement, switching it up with glandular forms can help them feel more energetic by introducing T_3 while lowering the T_4 dose to stop suppressing TSH.

Conventional medicine prefers synthetics, insisting that blood levels are more consistent. I do not treat blood levels; I focus on how a patient feels. Overtime, taking too much T_4 can cause osteoporosis. Too much T_3 can cause symptoms of high heart rate and nervous energy, so close communication with my patients is imperative to proper dosing of thyroid hormone.

My assessment of Doug is hypothalamus dysfunction with central hypothyroidism, hyperprolactinemia, and secondary hypogonadism.

Since Doug has been out of balance for a few years and living in a stressful family situation, we will need to support optimal hypothalamus function for at least a year, although I expect his prolactin to reach normal circadian levels within two to three months, his hypogonadism to resolve within three to four months and his central hypothyroidism to resolve within six to eight months.

Here's what Doug's healing plan looks like:

1. Hypothalamus support - I recommend Genesis Gold® 4gm of powder per fifty pounds of body weight plus 5gm of Sacred Seven® amino acids to be mixed with Genesis Gold® in water taken every morning at least fifteen minutes after taking thyroid hormone. While Sacred Seven® amino acids are in Genesis Gold®, I recommend adding more to address Doug's autoimmunity. It'll take months to lower his extremely high auto-thyroid antibodies.

2. Nutrition - Because Doug needs to lose weight and is currently consuming SAD, I recommend a liver cleanse diet for seven days followed by my insulin resistant diet. This should help him lose belly fat and lower his HGBA1C, which we will recheck in eight weeks.

3. Activity - Right now, we need to get Doug's energy up to get him moving. I recommend walking 30 minutes daily and to help slim his waist line - use a body hoop for fifteen minutes three times a week. A body hoop is a weighted adult sized hula hoop. They come in different sizes - the proper size is about waist height in diameter.

4. Sleep - I know that once we reset Doug's prolactin and with hypothalamic support, he will sleep better. In the meantime, I recommend using GABA 100-400mg in liquid form before bed. GABA is a calming neuropeptide that will help Doug relax and fall asleep. In liquid form, it works pretty quickly and can be taken at half dose if he wakes up in the middle of the night, which will help him to fall back to sleep. Of course, he's advised to sleep in a dark room and get off digital devices after dark.

5. Mindset - A healing mindset must be adopted yet Doug has lived in codependent relationships most of his life. He feels he needs to take care of everyone else and forgets to take care of himself. I recommend therapy for him and his family to learn better coping skills and for Doug to discover the root of his need to please.

6. To lower prolactin and reset circadian rhythm - I prescribe bromocryptine 2.5mg tablet to be inserted rectally first thing in the morning to raise dopamine and lower daytime prolactin. The extra Sacred Seven® hypothalamic amino acids will help Doug's hypothalamus make more dopamine as we wean him off bromocryptine. We will recheck his prolactin levels in a month.

7. Thyroid replacement therapy - I prescribe desiccated thyroid extract 2 grains (72mcg T_4/18mcg T_3) to be upon awakening and wait at least 30 minutes to eat. advise Doug to report excess T_3 symptoms of rapid heart rate or anxiety. He's to check BBT monthly, and we'll recheck his thyroid panel in 8-10 weeks to give his HPT axis time to adjust.

8. For androgenic hair loss - I recommend taking saw palmetto 360mg daily to help prevent excess dihydrotestosterone conversion and further hair loss.

Results

Just a few weeks later, Doug reports a big change in his energy and sleep patterns. "It feels like my body is waking up! I'm getting early morning erections again!" This is a great sign that his testosterone is peaking in the early morning and his receptor sites are more responsive to his sex hormones.

In Doug's case, he does not need supplemental testosterone therapy. Once we lower his prolactin and his thyroid hormone balances, he experiences greater testosterone effects. Of course, we focus on diet, exercise, and sleep habits, adjusting his plan according to his work schedule and when he has his children. His improved nutrition naturally shifts his family's diet as he learns to incorporate more vegetables, whole grains and legumes, less junk food and stops guzzling energy drinks. Besides, he doesn't need them anymore.

After a year of using nutraceutical hypothalamus support and the proper thyroid replacement, his autoantibodies drops. We're ready to see if his thyroid can start making its own hormones. So I recommend that he take one day a week off from the glandular. Over another year of slow weaning, Doug is able to get off thyroid hormone as he begins making adequate T_4 and T_3 with proper TSH response and has a normal BBT. Plus he's energetic, has lost body fat including his man boobs, increased his lean body mass, returned to his active lifestyle and started dating.

Chapter 6

Fatigue and Your Hypothalamus

Donna is a lovely lady who comes to me with adrenal fatigue and chronic fatigue syndrome. At 63, she's postmenopausal and has never taken hormones. She's been married for forty years, is a mother of three grown children and has four grandchildren. She's also an entrepreneur with a coaching business that focuses on women entrepreneurs. Her background is in business administration and she ran her husband's production company for over twenty years while raising the children. About fifteen years ago, she was diagnosed with chronic fatigue syndrome.

"So when did you have Epstein Barr virus?"

She looks at me surprised, "Why do you ask?"

"Because most people with chronic fatigue syndrome have a history of a virus that attacks the mitochondria."

"I've never been tested, but when my youngest was a teenager, she had mononucleosis. I spent two exhausting months nursing her back to health while running my coaching business and, of course, taking care of the household. I just never recovered from that stress. It took ten doctors before I was diagnosed with chronic fatigue syndrome."

"And when were you diagnosed with adrenal fatigue?"

"Right before going into menopause when I was 54."

"And you were never offered hormone replacement therapy?"

Donna shakes her head, "My grandmother had breast cancer, so my doctors didn't want to take the risk."

"So how did you manage your menopausal symptoms?"

"It was three years of hell - hot flashes, night sweats, insomnia, and brain fog. I just kept getting more and more fatigued. I never feel rested even if I take sleeping pills. I tried Chinese medicine and acupuncture, energy healing, functional medicine to treat my adrenal fatigue which would work for about six months, but then I would crash and nothing seemed to help. I haven't been able to have sex in years. It's too painful. And I'm peeing all the time and it hurts. I can't tell you how many doctors have prescribed antibiotics for UTIs but it doesn't help the constant need to go to the bathroom."

It's not unusual for healthcare providers to avoid offering HRT to a woman with a family history of hormone fed cancer. Yet, every case is individual. Even women with breast cancer should be given the option for some relief of their symptoms. That may mean botanicals or vaginal estrogen, and at least hypothalamic support. Menopause makes pre-existing conditions so much worse. Your body needs sex steroids for healthy metabolism, cell rejuvenation and strong immunity.

Typical of people with adrenal issues, Donna describes herself as an anxious person. She gets stressed easily. Her go-to remedy when she was younger was to exercise, which is a great way to manage stress. A constantly firing HPA axis will eventually lead to adrenal issues. Aerobic exercise helps burn off adrenaline and cortisol while regulating the HPA axis. Except once Donna became infected with Epstein Barr virus, her mitochondria could no longer produce the energy she needed to run off her stress.

"I've tried to use magnesium to calm down but whenever I take it, I get more anxious, my heart races, and I can't sleep. I don't know what to do."

Donna is describing a paradoxical reaction - meaning the opposite reaction than expected. I suspect that since her hypothalamus has been dysfunctional for at least two decades, her detox pathways are not functioning properly and she has a mineral deficiency. So yes, she probably needs magnesium, but her cells cannot use it properly causing excitatory rather than neuro-calming effects.

The importance of the Physical Exam

I try to physically examine all of my patients. In this age of telemedicine, it's not always possible, yet relying on the findings of another practitioner is dicey. Plus the examining table is a great setting for teaching patients how to examine their own bodies.

Upon examining Donna, she appears to be pretty healthy. She has a slender build with fine bone structure which puts her at greater risk for osteoporosis. We will definitely evaluate bone loss with a DEXA scan and urine crosslinks test. She has no thyroid enlargement. Her breast exam reveals no nodularity and bilateral implants that appear to be intact without contractures. Donna is happy with her implants and has been getting regular breast imaging. I teach her full breast exam as it's important, especially with implants, that she knows the difference between her implants and her normal glandular tissue.

I use the clock to teach self-breast exam. Mammary glands are located at 10-12 o'clock on the right breast and 12-2 o'clock on the left breast. From 3-9 o'clock is normal fibrous tissue that holds the breast to the chest wall. Women with fibrocystic condition may notice little more prominent fibrous tissue and sometimes tender cysts. What you're looking for are very hard lumps that do not move within the breast. Normal glandular tissue feels like a contracted muscle. Suspicious breast lumps can be as hard as your elbow. Any dimpling of the breast tissue may indicate a mass that is pulling on the skin. Normal breast lumps like cysts and mammary glands float in the breast tissue, not rooted down like malignant masses.

The lymph nodes that drain the breasts lie under the breast in a semi-circle and extend into the axillae (armpit). They're typically not palpable unless inflamed. Unlike the round lymph nodes in your neck, these are more like flat beans. It is not unusual to feel prominent tender nodes right where the underwire of your bra presses. Switching to no-wire support can help relieve the pressure, as will gentle massage and taking off your bra at least overnight.

I also check for nipple discharge using a white tissue to blot and check color. A small amount of white or clear discharge is normal. Any other color is abnormal. You should examine your breasts monthly, after your period or anytime of the month once you're menopausal. In my practice, most of my well-taught patients find their own breast lumps because they know what they're looking for.

Once a woman is postmenopausal without hormone replacement therapy, her breast tissue diminishes considerably. So, Donna may notice changes in her breasts with more prominent glandular tissue if she decides to start bioidentical hormone replacement therapy. Initial breast fullness and tenderness is common when first initiating HRT and usually calms down after the first couple of months.

I notice that Donna has a diastasis, a separation of the abdominal rectus muscles. We're all born with one, which is why babies have little Buddha bellies. By the time a child has been walking for at least a year, the diastasis closes as the abdominal rectus muscles come together. When a woman is pregnant, her rectus muscles naturally separate to accommodate her expanding uterus. This normal diastasis of pregnancy usually closes in the first few months postpartum. Women who've had multiple pregnancies or pregnancies close together may not heal up their diastasis. Donna has a two centimeter diastasis from just below her sternum down to her umbilicus, extending about halfway to her pubic bone.

I teach Donna some exercises that she can do to strengthen her abdominal rectus muscles. She may not be able to close her diastasis this long after her pregnancies, but it will help prevent further herniation. I instruct her to lie on her back with a folded towel around her waist. She crosses her arms and holds onto the ends of the towel as if cinching her waist. Then I ask her to raise her feet 2-3 inches off the ground while lifting her head slightly and looking down towards her feet. Unlike sit-ups, this exercise strengthens the length of the abdominal rectus muscles. She is to hold that position for three to five seconds and do at least 10 to 20 repetitions daily.

When I was being trained as a nurse practitioner, we, students, would examine one another. My student partner noticed that I had a diastasis. It had been over a year since I gave birth and thin like Donna, I had lost my baby weight shortly after birth, but my waist was one inch larger. The instructor taught me this very same exercise which closed my diastasis within a couple of months.

On her pelvic exam, I note that Donna has a very atrophic vulva and vagina and a prolapsed urethra - no wonder sex hurts. Vaginal atrophy is extreme thinning of the vulvar and vaginal tissues due to lack of estrogen. I'm not surprised that Donna has mild urethral prolapse. The urethra is the tiny opening leading to the bladder which is normally tucked into the upper vaginal opening. When it's prolapsed, the urethra is prominent and red as the inner surface is folded outward. The bladder and urethra are also estrogen dependent. It's no wonder Donna is complaining of urinary frequency.

With vaginal atrophy, the tissue appears pale, not the normal pink. Blood vessels are visible through the atrophied epithelium, giving the vaginal walls a red eye look. The tissue also feels thinner as there's an absence of the normal rugation or natural folds of the vagina.

A healthy well estrogenized vagina has multiple rugations that allow it to encompass coitus and childbirth. The thick epithelial layers produce more than enough lubrication to keep the natural microflora of the vagina, lactobacillus acidophilus, thriving as they feed off vaginal cell glycogen.

Donna needs topical vaginal estrogen to rejuvenate the atrophy and make intercourse and urination comfortable. Estrogen applied directly into the vagina works much faster than systemic estrogen and is very safe. Even before we do testing to determine how Donna is actually metabolizing her hormones and to make sure that it's safe to give her hormones with her family history of breast cancer, she can start healing her vagina.

I prescribe estriol vaginal cream to be applied nightly for at least eight weeks to help thicken the vaginal epithelium and increase natural lubrication. She will also notice an improvement in her frequent urination as estriol will help heal her chronic urethritis.

Unfortunately most healthcare providers assume a urinary tract infection (UTI) when a menopausal woman complains of urinary frequency. Most of the time, it's the lack of estrogen that causes an inflamed urethra, a weak bladder neck, a constant need to urinate and stress incontinence. Of course, if there's a pathogenic bacterial overgrowth in the urine, it needs to be treated, but prescribing antibiotics based on symptoms alone puts the patient's gut at risk and does not address the atrophy.

I also note on Donna's exam that she has some sarcopenia - loss of muscle tissue. Now she's a slender postmenopausal woman, so I expect a little bit of loosening up in her triceps area but all of her muscles are quite thin. And she doesn't have upper body strength, which is affecting her ability to pick up her grandbabies. We want to get Donna stronger and help build up her bones because she's at high risk for osteoporosis. Slender Caucasian women have a higher risk of osteoporosis when they lose their sex hormones. Weight resistance exercise is critical to build muscle and bone. Plus, we will need to replace all of her bone building hormones.

But first, we must address her chronic fatigue syndrome before she's going to be able to effectively exercise.

Donna is my typical patient with multiple diagnoses who has not found relief in either conventional or complementary medicine. Yes, they provide symptom relief, but remember that's downstream medicine. What Donna needs is upstream medicine.

So, we're going to get to the root of her issues. And we are going back in time to when it all began, which is probably much farther back than she realizes. And we will focus treatment on her hypothalamus.

CFS and Mitochondrial Dysfunction

Let's start with Donna's chronic fatigue syndrome because at the heart of CFS is mitochondrial dysfunction. Mitochondria are tiny cellular organelles that produce energy and are known as the cell powerhouse. Every cell in your body has hundreds of mitochondria. Your most active cells like neurons and muscles have many more. If the mitochondria do not work, cells die. Mitochondrial dysfunction means the cell powerhouses are producing energy at minimal capacity.

Chronic fatigue syndrome is characterized by damage to the mitochondria and it affects the mitochondria in all the cells of the body, including the brain, muscles, and vital organs. Some days are better while some days are worse. Donna cannot overdo it or she'll wipe herself out for days. Even mental exertion can cause extreme fatigue for days. CFS can be very debilitating, sometimes debilitating enough to not be able to work. You just don't have the get up and go, and you can also have brain fog and depression because you just aren't producing enough energy in the brain.

Donna's CFS complicates her menopause and vice versa. Her CFS got worse as she entered menopause. That's because estrogen helps keep insulin receptors healthy. Mitochondria need glucose to generate energy. When glucose cannot get into the cells due to insulin receptor issues, then the mitochondria have to use vital cell fatty acids to produce energy and that depletes vital nutrients and creates more cellular waste. No wonder Donna has paradoxical reactions.

Chronic Fatigue Syndrome affects the muscles and brain and is often referred to as myalgic encephalomyelitis/chronic fatigue syndrome (ME/CFS).

While there's no test for ME/CFS, there are guidelines to help diagnose the condition. First, healthcare providers have to rule out other issues, so these tests are used to assess for other underlying causes of fatigue:

- Complete blood cell count to rule out anemia (Donna is not anemic)
- Chemistries including electrolytes, renal, and liver function tests (all within normal limits for Donna)
- Thyroid function tests to rule out hypothyroidism (Donna has healthy TSH:T_4/T_3)
- C-reactive protein - a measurement of cardiovascular inflammation (no sign of cardiovascular inflammation for Donna)

- Erythrocyte sedimentation rate to rule out systemic inflammation (Donna has a slight elevation of ESR)

- Creatine kinase - a measurement of muscle breakdown (Donna has a moderate elevation which explains her sarcopenia)

According to the National Academy of Medicine, diagnosis of ME/CFS requires the presence of the following three symptoms for more than six months, and the intensity of the symptoms should be moderate or severe for at least 50% of the time:

- Fatigue: A noticeable decrease or impairment in the ability of a patient to engage in activities that they enjoyed before the onset of the illness, with this impairment continuing for more than 6 months and associated with new-onset severe fatigue, unrelated to exertion, and not relieved by rest.

- Post-exertional malaise (PEM): Patients experience worsening symptoms and function after exposure to physical or cognitive stressors that were previously well-tolerated.

- Unrefreshing sleep: Patients feel tired after a night's sleep.

Plus one of these symptoms:

- Cognitive impairment - Problems with the thought or executive function, worsened by exertion, effort, stress or time pressure.

- Orthostatic intolerance - Worsening of symptoms upon assuming and maintaining an upright posture. Symptoms are improved, although not necessarily eliminated by lying back down or elevating the feet.

Many viruses have been studied as potential causes of CFS; however, no definitive causal relation has been determined. Some people infected with Epstein-Barr virus, Ross River virus, Coxiella burnetii, Giardia and

SARS-COV-19 have developed criteria for CFS, but not all individuals with CFS have had these infections. Studies have observed alterations in the functioning of natural killer (NK) cells and a decreased response of T-cells to certain specific antigens.

Environmental factors have also been suspected as a trigger for CFS; however, no specific factors have been identified.

Since Donna's extreme fatigue followed exposure to her daughter's mononucleosis, we can assume that Epstein Barr Virus (EBV) may have triggered her ME/CFS. While over 85% of adults have antibodies against EBV and not all develop ME/CFS, I have found in the majority of my ME/CFS patients that they have very high viral loads of EBV.

EBV can be detected by these tests:

- **Viral capsid antigen (VCA)**: Anti-VCA IgM appears early in EBV infection and usually disappears within four to six weeks. Anti-VCA IgG appears in the acute phase of EBV infection, peaks at two to four weeks after onset, declines slightly then persists for the rest of a person's life. Anti-VCA IgG over 20 is positive for past infection. People with high viral loads or reactivated EBV have IgG levels in the hundreds.

- **Early antigen (EA)** Anti-EA IgG appears in the acute phase of illness and generally falls to undetectable levels after three to six months. In 80% of people, detection of antibody to EA is a sign of active infection.

- **EBV nuclear antigen (EBNA)** Antibody to EBNA, determined by the standard immunofluorescent test, is not seen in the acute phase of EBV infection but slowly appears two to four months after onset of symptoms and persists for the rest of a person's life.

Donna's VCA IgG is over 600 and her anti-EA IgG is elevated as well, so we will focus on helping her immune system manage EBV more effectively. Supporting her hypothalamus with Genesis Gold® will further help her condition by optimizing her immune function so her T-cells help eradicate EBV.

Assessing Bone Health

Donna is surprised at her height, claiming she's lost over an inch. "I used to be 5'7"!" Bone loss in the vertebrae can cause significant loss of height.

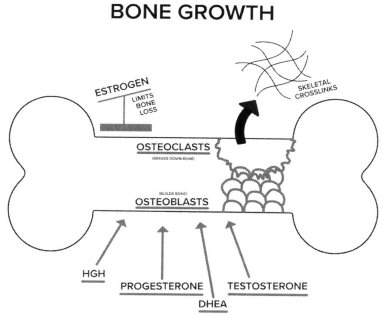

BONE GROWTH

D. MARAGOPOULOS © 2023

Two types of cells - osteocytes- are responsible for bone formation. Osteoblasts form the protein matrix in which minerals are deposited. Osteoblasts are stimulated by growth factors including DHEA, testosterone, progesterone and growth hormone. Osteoclasts eat away old bone so new bone can be laid down. Your skeleton today is not the same bone as your skeleton of last year. That's why checking bone density by dexa scan reflects past habits and health. Checking skeletal crosslinks in the urine or blood reflects active bone loss. Estrogen controls the rate of osteoclast activity.

My concern with treating Donna's osteoporosis is her getting enough bone building minerals in light of her paradoxical reaction to magnesium.

Magnesium usually has a calming effect on the nervous system, muscles, and the heart. Symptoms of magnesium deficiency are muscle cramps, weakness, anxiety, irritability, gastrointestinal spasms, headache. Too little magnesium at the neuromuscular junction of the heart can cause arrhythmias. Yet, Donna is complaining of heart palpitations and anxiety when she takes magnesium.

Like all minerals, magnesium is dependent upon other electrolytes - calcium, sodium, potassium, chloride - to interact with cell membranes. Magnesium is also highly dependent on intracellular glutathione - a powerful antioxidant produced by the liver and involved in many vital cell functions.

Three conditionally essential amino acids, glycine, cysteine, and glutamic acid combine to form glutathione (GSH). Essential amino acids are those you must consume as your body doesn't make them. Conditionally essential amino acids are those your body makes naturally but can become depleted during illness, injury or high physiological stress. Glutathione production is very dependent upon your diet. Consuming enough protein and sulfur rich foods like cruciferous vegetables, alliums, and eggs can help provide your body with enough conditionally essential amino acids. Omega-3 fatty acids found in fatty fish help reduce inflammation by combating oxidation and can help increase glutathione reserves. Phytonutrients from a variety of colorful produce helps increase GSH stores to reduce potential paradoxical reactions.

Donna's chemistry panel is within normal limits, which is not surprising. Cellular mineral deficiencies often do not show in the blood serum as the cardiovascular system needs the main electrolytes to stay within narrow parameters to properly function. Your hypothalamus insures your heart functions for your survival so electrolyte imbalances are an ominous sign of serious hypothalamus dysfunction, kidney disease or parathyroid disorders.

There are four pea-sized parathyroid glands located behind the butterfly shaped thyroid, one on each lobe. The parathyroid glands have one job - to regulate blood calcium levels in a very tight range between 8.5 and 10.5. When calcium levels are too low, these glands produce parathyroid hormone which pulls calcium from your bones and influences the intestinal lining to become more efficient at absorbing calcium normally found in the diet. Too much parathyroid hormone can cause osteoporosis.

I only check parathyroid hormone levels if blood calcium levels are high or if a person has osteoporosis at a very young age. I expect some bone loss in Donna since she's postmenopausal, Caucasian and of slender build. Plus, she's never been offered hormones to prevent menopausal bone loss. Estrogen helps prevent excess bone turnover. So, I order a bone crosslinks test either through blood or urine which can determine if Donna is actively losing bone.

I also order a dexa scan to determine if she has existing bone loss. A dexa scan is an X-ray that measures skeletal calcium. The most accurate dexa scans are done on the hip which is the most prone to fracture and the lumbar spine which will show vertebral height loss. Sometimes I get patients referred for hormone consultation from dentists who notice bone loss in their jaw. Dexa scans of the heel or wrist are not as accurate as the hip and spine.

Donna's dexa scan shows osteoporosis and her crosslinks is elevated, meaning she's still actively losing bone. Donna needs estrogen to stop the bone loss.

After stopping active bone loss, building bone requires three things - bone growth promoting hormones, adequate bone building nutrients, and weight resistance exercise to stimulate bone growth.

Being postmenopausal, Donna's FSH is high which indicates her pituitary is not getting enough estrogen. It was probably much higher in early menopause as typically FSH goes down after the pituitary gives up on the ovaries ever producing estrogen again. Donna's LH is high too because she is not making any progesterone, which she will need to help build bone.

I measure Donna's other bone building hormones - testosterone, DHEA, and determine her growth hormone levels by measuring IgF-1 - all of which are low as expected at her postmenopausal age.

Donna needs HRT not only to help reverse her osteoporosis, but to alleviate her postmenopausal symptoms, prevent dementia, and help heal her mitochondria.

Donna also needs hypothalamic support as the ventromedial nuclei regulates bone metabolism. The hypothalamus hormone orexin is critical in regulating skeletal homeostasis and bone mass, while leptin inhibits bone formation through the sympathetic nervous system.

Since Donna has osteoporosis, she needs to pay particular attention to her diet and may need supplementation. We calculate her ideal lean body mass at 100 pounds (although she's ten pounds light) and estimate her minimal protein needs at 50 gm per day. Her vitamin D levels are low at 27, so she will need supplementation to ensure dietary minerals are deposited properly in her bones. Plus, vitamin D enhances hormone receptor site function.

It is recommended that women over the age of 50 and men over 70 get 1200mg of elemental calcium daily, mostly from their diet as it's difficult for the body to absorb more than 500mg of supplemental calcium. Yet, less than 10% of women and less than 25% of men get enough calcium daily.

Calcium supplements are derived from bones, shells, and algae. While calcium citrate is more absorbable than other forms of calcium salts, it only contains 21% elemental calcium, meaning is usable by the human body. Taking calcium with food in dosages of 500 mg or less increases absorption. The absorption rate for calcium is about 20 to 30 percent. Foods such as spinach, rhubarb and wheat bran can decrease calcium absorption. Calcium can interfere with absorption of iron, zinc, bisphosphonates and tetracycline. Calcium absorption also requires adequate doses of vitamin D.

Many nutrients play a role in bone health - protein, calcium, magnesium, phosphorus, boron, potassium, vitamin D and Vitamin K. A healthy diet with lots of fruits, vegetables, legumes, nuts, seeds, and lean proteins provides most of the essential nutrients needed to keep bones healthy.

HRT and Cancer

Before talking about HRT, we have a frank conversation about the risk of cancer. In Donna's case, it is her paternal grandmother who had breast cancer in her eighties, but died of heart disease. She has no other relatives with breast or ovarian cancer. I am particularly interested in any relatives that may have had mutated BRCA genes.

Breast Cancer genes 1 and 2 produce proteins that help repair damaged DNA. Everyone has two copies of each of these genes—one copy inherited from each parent. BRCA1 and BRCA2 are sometimes called tumor suppressor genes. If BRCA genes have harmful mutations, cancer can develop - most notably breast and ovarian cancer, but also several additional types of cancer. People who have inherited a harmful variant in BRCA1 and BRCA2 also tend to develop cancer at younger ages than people who do not have such a variant. A harmful variant in BRCA1 or BRCA2 can be inherited from either parent.

Donna is not at a great risk of breast cancer but we will check how she metabolizes estrogen by looking at her estriol to estrone ratios - particularly 2OH estrone and 16OH estrone. Postmenopausal women tend to have low protective 2OH estrone compared to inflammatory 16OH estrone, but her ratio will determine how much her diet and lifestyle need to be changed and if she needs additional supplementation. Donna is already slender and does not abuse alcohol which is great because obesity and excessive alcohol intake increases inflammatory 16OH estrone. If necessary, adding EPA, flax lignans and especially DIM can help convert estradiol into protective 2OH estrone.

Donna's 2OH to 16OH estrogen ratio is low, so we will start with 200mg of DIM daily.

Even though Donna's testosterone levels are low and testosterone can promote bone growth, I'm going to recommend starting with estrogen, progesterone and DHEA which can convert into testosterone. I want to see how she does on estrogen and progesterone to relieve her symptoms.

Administering testosterone is never my first choice for hormone replacement therapy in menopausal women. Unlike many healthcare providers, especially those who promote pellets, I do not prescribe high doses of testosterone. I am not a fan of pellets, which only provide testosterone and estrogen but not progesterone for hormone replacement therapy. Excessive testosterone increases small particle LDL and can cause mood changes. And while testosterone does convert into estrogen, there's no controlling the conversion.

Testosterone is often utilized by practitioners to increase a woman's libido, but in my clinical experience working with hormonally challenged women for over 30 years, I've rarely had to use testosterone for libido in women. If we get her estrogen levels where they need to be with enough progesterone to open up estrogen receptors, most women's libidos are restored. Besides postmenopausal women tend to have higher testosterone levels because theca cells produce testosterone for much longer after menopause, but it's not converted into adequate amounts of estrogen, hence, the increase in facial hair in postmenopausal women.

Estrogen is the hormone of libido for the majority of women. While testosterone affects female libido, it does not increase desire, arousal or orgasmic potential like estrogen. I've found that the majority of my patients' libidos and sexual responsiveness respond well to estrogen and progesterone. In the rare patient, maybe one out of 10, I will add testosterone replacement. If their osteoporosis is severe and we're not able to raise testosterone with DHEA replacement, then I will add testosterone but in very small doses. High dose testosterone can cause tendon ruptures in women.

As for Donna's low IgF-1, indicating low human growth hormone levels, I still start with sex steroid hormone replacement and DHEA before adding amino acid precursors that can increase human growth hormone production. If that doesn't work, I may prescribe human growth hormone by injection but the majority of the time growth hormone increases naturally when the hypothalamus is supported and sex steroids and DHEA are replaced at adequate levels.

I always have my female patients take a three day break from their BHRT every month, whether they're menstruating or not, in order to clear their receptor sites so that they can use a lot less hormones. Many of my patients will say that they used hormones before and it worked great for the first six months but after that they didn't feel anything. That's because their receptor sites never got a break and they became desensitized to the hormones. Their healthcare providers probably had to keep changing the type of hormones, the delivery system, and the dose of hormones when if they would have prescribed a break from the beginning, the patient wouldn't have become hormonally resistant. In the worst cases of severe hormone depletion, a woman has forty weeks before she must take a break. Your hypothalamus does not recognize you being on hormones every single day without taking a break for more than the length of a full term pregnancy. It takes 72 hours to clear the receptor sites.

I prefer to avoid oral routes of administering hormones. Except progesterone, the other steroid hormones are best used sublingually (under the tongue) or transdermally (through the skin). Since steroid hormones are made of fat molecules, I have my compounders use a liposomal base for best absorption. For female BHRT, application on the inner thigh is the best place for absorption and longer action.

After testing, Donna agrees to try BHRT. But before we initiate BHRT, we need to evaluate Donna's adrenal glands.

Is adrenal fatigue real?

Originally, some healthcare providers did a saliva test on Donna and determined she had adrenal fatigue. I don't necessarily do saliva tests anymore. In the first few years of my integrative practice, I did run 24 urine and saliva tests and found ultimately that my assessment of the patient through a thorough history, physical exam and certain blood tests gave me the information I needed to determine endocrinological functioning.

One of the reasons I stopped doing saliva testing as a way to measure adrenal function is that I had a patient that I suspected had adrenal dysfunction. When her saliva test came back, it showed a high spike of cortisol in the middle of the day, during the time she usually felt low.

Clearly something stressed her. In fact, she started taking her saliva test, collecting saliva first thing in the morning and at noon. Then she went on a hike and broke her ankle. But before going to the ER, she collected her midafternoon saliva. Of course, having an injury like that caused a cortisol spike. So it matters what's going on that day. We can't control all the stress that may cause a spike and not be reflective of day to day adrenal function.

Measuring sulfated DHEA helps me determine cortisol because DHEA naturally follows cortisol.

When you're experiencing a stressor, your adrenals are supposed to act in a certain way. The stressor does not have to be life threatening, but according to how much stress you feel is how your adrenals react in the face of a life threatening stressor like a tiger is chasing you.

The Stress Response

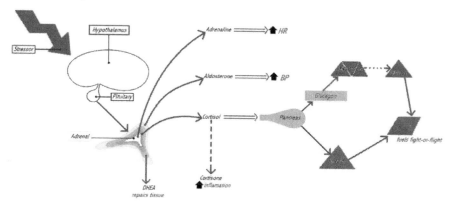

Copyright D Maragopoulos 2016

Immediately you get an adrenaline surge forcing an elevation in your heart rate and your blood pressure, so you can get away from danger. That surge of adrenaline tells the hypothalamus that you need more cortisol produced.

Your hypothalamus stimulates your pituitary gland to release ACTH which stimulates your adrenals to produce cortisol. Cortisol stimulates your pancreas to release glucagon. Glucagon is the opposite of insulin - it stimulates the release of glycogen, which is stored sugar, from your liver and your muscles. Now, your cells can make enough energy to run away from the tiger.

DHEA production follows cortisol. If your cortisol levels have been high, your DHEA levels will be high as well. DHEA helps you to metabolize protein and fat to repair the damage from the fight or flight. Your blood pressure is sustained by a hormone called aldosterone. Aldosterone controls salt/water balance keeping potassium in the blood and pulling water and sodium out through the kidneys.

If you don't produce enough aldosterone, you're going to have orthostatic hypotension, meaning when you stand up really quickly, you feel dizzy because your blood pressure bottoms out. I measure aldosterone function in a patient by checking their blood pressure after lying down for a few minutes, then immediately standing them up and checking their blood pressure again. If they have normal aldosterone production, their blood pressure should go up 10 to 20 points. If they have poor aldosterone production, their blood pressure stays the same or worse goes down - that's orthostatic hypotension.

Adrenal fatigue can affect aldosterone production too. Donna's orthostatic blood pressure drops, another sign of adrenal dysfunction and ME/CFS.

Checking DHEA-S, which is the active form of DHEA, tells me how much cortisol the adrenal glands are producing. Checking unconjugated DHEA tells me how much adrenal reserve there is. Donna has very low DHEA-S and unconjugated DHEA.

Cortisol gets converted into cortisone, which is anti-inflammatory. After experiencing stress, there might be some inflammation from the fight or flight. Except if you don't really have to run away from danger, then not only do you have too much glucose floating around which is inflammatory but all that extra cortisol is converted into too much cortisone. Cortisol and cortisone are catabolic, meaning they break down tissue.

Let's say you're really worried about something - a loved one, bills, your health, etc. Overtime, the high levels of stress hormones eat away at your tissues - muscles, bones, intestines, skin, hair. If you've ever had to use cortisone cream for a rash, it's recommended that you wash it off your hands because not only will cortisone reduce the inflamed rash but it will thin the skin of your fingertips.

Primary adrenal insufficiency is known as Addison's disease. This rare condition may occur at any age when the adrenal glands are damaged usually by an autoimmune attack following an infection.

Secondary adrenal insufficiency starts when the hypothalamus does not stimulate the pituitary gland to make enough ACTH, so the adrenal glands don't make enough cortisol.

Symptoms of adrenal insufficiency may include:

- Weakness
- Fatigue
- Dizziness
- Muscle aches
- Lack of appetite
- Nausea
- Vomiting
- Diarrhea
- Weight loss
- Fluid loss (dehydration)
- Low blood pressure
- Low sugar levels
- Irregular or no menstrual periods
- Dark skin (Addison's disease only)

Bluish-black color around the nipples, mouth, rectum, scrotum, or vagina (Addison's disease only)

The gold standard test for adrenal insufficiency is an ACTH stimulation test. This test measures your adrenal glands' response after you're given an injection of synthetic ACTH. Adrenal insufficiency is conclusive if one hour after the injection, the adrenal glands only produce very low levels of cortisol.

Although adrenal fatigue is not an accepted medical diagnosis, it is believed that after long periods of stress, the adrenal glands can get worn out. Some patients misdiagnosed with adrenal fatigue actually have postural orthostatic tachycardia syndrome (POTS), a surprisingly common condition, where your heart races, your blood pressure lowers and you have no energy. POTS is often rooted in hypothalamus dysfunction.

Normal adrenal production of cortisol is high with spikes from 8am to 2pm, after eating, and during intense activity, then drops naturally in the late afternoon and finally surges slightly at dinner time with very low production at night.

What I see in my practice are stressed out hormonally challenged people whose adrenal function is not circadian. They use caffeine and sugar to keep their energy up in the afternoon which stimulates adrenal cortisol production not allowing normal rest. They don't have the best sleep habits, so they continue to stimulate adrenal cortisol production at night with too much screen time, watching fearful news and stressing themselves out.

Your adrenals are meant to function for your lifetime, naturally fading with old age. We were not meant to be living with constant stress, working long hours and not resting. Stress reactions are learned behaviors and can be modified but it takes practice.

Donna's DHEA-S is low even for her age and her reserve as measured by her unconjugated DHEA is even lower.

When your hypothalamus is supported nutraceutically, it helps to regulate adrenal function in more natural rhythms, allowing your stress response to calm down and preserving adrenal function.

My assessment of Donna is hypothalamus dysfunction with myalgic encephalopathy/chronic fatigue syndrome, complicated by postmenopausal osteoporosis and adrenal insufficiency.

Since Donna has been out of balance for nearly twenty years, we will need to support optimal hypothalamus function for at least two years, although I suspect she will experience an increase in energy and decrease in active bone loss over the next few months, and increase in bone density over the next few years.

Here's what Donna's healing plan looks like:

1. Hypothalamus support - I recommend Genesis Gold® 4gm of powder mixed in water per fifty pounds of body weight taken every morning at least fifteen minutes before eating breakfast. Supporting her hypothalamus with Genesis Gold® will help heal her over activated HPA axis, improve mitochondrial function and mitigate menopausal symptoms like insomnia, plus the plant derived micronutrients help to improve hormone metabolism.

2. Nutrition - I recommend my DMAR® Nutritional Path to Wellness - a modified version of the Mediterranean diet with formulas to calculate protein, fat and carbohydrate needs. Donna needs to eat more protein to maintain and build up her LBM. I recommend at least 20g of protein per meal. I also recommend that she incorporate sea salt into her diet which will help her orthostatic hypotension. I advise that she try to consume 800-1000mg of calcium from her diet daily.

3. Activity - I recommend mild aerobic activity until she regains her energy. And add weight resistance exercises a few times per week. Weight resistance exercise is crucial to stimulating bone growth. Plus, stretching every day to prevent joint injuries.

4. Sleep - Besides sleeping in the dark, I strongly recommend that Donna take a break from watching the news or anything stimulating before bed. Plus, I recommend a relaxing bedtime routine like a hot bath and meditation to calm her nervous system.

5. Mindset - Donna actually has a pretty healthy mindset but she's better at taking care of others than herself. And she could use some support, so I invite her into my Hormone Healing Circle to provide easily accessible virtual support during the first year of her healing journey.

6. For mitochondrial repair - I recommend a special blend of phospho-glycolipids to help heal her cell membranes which will allow mitochondrial cofactors to get into the cells and increase energy production. Mitochondrial cofactors include lipoic acid, and activated B1, B2, B3, B5 vitamins. Adding homeopathic immune support against EBV will help her T-cells recognize EBV and help prevent further mitochondrial damage.

7. For osteoporosis and postmenopausal atrophy - I recommend;

- Vaginal estriol cream 1mg/gm, apply one gram nightly for at least six weeks before reducing to every other night for a few weeks, then once a week or as needed for urinary frequency or coital discomfort.

- Estradiol tablets 0.5mg SL (under the tongue) daily - take a three day break per month. Estrogen will help stop bone loss.

- Micronized Progesterone 100mg capsules before bed to help her sleep - we can switch to transdermal preparation once her sleep improves - take a three day break per month along with estradiol. Progesterone can help build bone.

- DIM 200mg daily to help her metabolize estrogen more safely.

- DHEA 12.5mg SL six mornings per week to help build bone.

- Vitamin D 10,000IUs daily taken with fat for best absorption.

- Once her paradoxical reactions diminish, we will add supplemental calcium if she cannot get enough in her diet.

8. For paradoxical reactions - I recommend trace minerals to provide necessary cofactors and to avoid high dose mineral supplementation. Omega 3 fatty acids 2000mg twice daily to help increase GSH reserve. Increase consumption of asparagus, avocado, spinach and green beans which are rich sources of GHS, as well as brassica vegetables and strive for colorful veggies and fruit for increased phytonutrients.

Results

Within the first month, Donna reports that her sleep has definitely improved which helps with her daytime fatigue. Her urinary frequency ceased and sex is much more comfortable. She's doing well on BHRT with DIM helping to mitigate breast tenderness and fluid retention.

After eight weeks, we recheck her crosslinks to determine if her estrogen dose is adequate to stop bone loss. While her crosslinks test showed significantly less bone loss, it wasn't low enough, so we increase estradiol to 0.75mg daily. She's tolerating her three day hormone break well, although she notices her brain isn't quite as sharp on her days off BHRT.

Eight weeks after increasing her estradiol dose, her crosslinks test indicates no active bone loss. Donna has so much more energy that she's able to do both daily aerobic exercise and weight resistance three times a week and has noticeable improvement in muscle mass. Her weight is up by five pounds but her body fat remains the same, indicating an increase in lean body mass.

After a year of consistent exercise, improved diet, BHRT and nutraceuticals, Donna's dexa scan shows an increase in bone calcium. She's ecstatic that she's regained a half inch of height too. She's on her way to reversing her osteoporosis.

Donna is consistent in supporting her hypothalamus with Genesis Gold® and finds out that taking a little bit extra on her days off BHRT helps with her brain fog. She thrives in the Hormone Healing Circle, appreciating the group support and accountability to her healing goals.

Chapter 7

Neurological Disorders, Addiction and Your Hypothalamus

Richard is a 58 year old gentleman who consults with me for long covid. Since contracting covid over a year ago, he's been exhausted with significant brain fog, depression and weakness.

"I can't work anymore. Before getting covid, I was able to function. Now everything is getting worse."

A contractor by trade, he injured his back in his early thirties. Lumbar surgery did not relieve his back pain and he became dependent on opiates. Richard has a long history of drug use from his teen years and has been in rehab seven times. Raised by an alcoholic abusive father and molested by his priest, Richard also had a significant history of adverse childhood experiences. Adverse childhood experiences or ACEs have been correlated with many chronic illnesses - depression, diabetes, cardiovascular disease and predication to substance abuse.

Richard's condition is complicated by multiple sclerosis. He was diagnosed shortly before his back injury when he complained of visual disturbances and a brain MRI revealed demyelination of his optic nerve. Over the past two decades, he's experienced more symptoms including sensory loss, heat intolerance, muscle cramping and depression. Like most MS patients, Richard has had symptomatic episodes over the years that have affected different body parts.

"I've managed my MS but since covid, it's gotten worse."

Multiple sclerosis is an autoimmune demyelinating disease that affects over 2.3 million individuals worldwide. Auto reactive immune cells attack myelin and axons of central nervous system neurons, leading to destructive lesions in the spinal cord and brain. Hypothalamic dysfunction is common in chronic inflammatory diseases like MS and the hypothalamus is frequently affected by MS containing many active demyelinated lesions.

The etiology of MS is unknown but toxins, viruses, lack of vitamin D, substance abuse and childhood trauma have been implicated. Nearly one third of MS patients will become significantly disabled.

I ask about his toxic exposures and discover that he lived in Africa for a few years around puberty.

"I'm an army brat. My father was stationed all over the world. But it's interesting that you ask because I recently got in touch with some of the kids at the base in Ethiopia. All the women have breast cancer. I'm the only one with MS, but the other guys have been dealing with health issues too." With more questioning, I find out that the men all have various autoimmune conditions. And the army discovered arsenic in the well water that all these pubescent children drank. We will test Richard for heavy metal toxicity.

Since his MS was progressing slowly, Richard tried to avoid immune modulating treatments. Now he needs help.

At his age, I suspect Richard is also in andropause. He has had significant erectile dysfunction for years and admits that he's noticed a decrease in morning erections over the past decade which is a sign of declining testosterone. He also complains of his sleep being interrupted by nocturia a few times at night and difficulty initiating urination. As men's testosterone lowers, their prostate enlarges causing pressure on the bladder neck.

Studies show that the hormonal decline and hypothalamic dysregulation at the change of life can worsen MS pathology. Andropause appears to contribute to immunosenescence, an age-associated decline in function of both the adaptive and innate immune systems.

So, we need to address Richard's declining hormones to help him recover from the long-term damage of covid and prevent progression of disability from multiple sclerosis.

Richard's physical exam

In my physical examination of Richard, I note his thinness, which is typical of patients with multiple sclerosis. Weight loss is common in MS due to sarcopenia or muscle loss from lack of adequate nerve stimulation. His body also shows signs of low testosterone with flat deltoids.

His rectal exam reveals a slightly enlarged prostate without nodularity which may be causing some of his nocturia. His testicles are small, which suggests that he has not been producing enough testosterone for a while. He's showing signs of aging with some loosening of his skin.

Most significant is Richard's neurological examination. He has an intentional tremor. His gait shows mild stumbling and he has some weakness of both of his quadriceps. He also has mild paraesthesia of his fingers and hands in a glove distribution as well as his toes and feet in a sock distribution.

My plan for Richard is to definitely support his hypothalamus. I've found in other patients with neurological conditions that hypothalamic support is critical to diminishing symptoms of fatigue, anxiety, depression and brain fog. Hypothalamic support helps to diminish neurological symptoms in long COVID as well.

We also need to work on trying to repair his myelin. Now, traditionally, medicine does not believe that nerves can be repaired after being damaged. But certain hormones do stimulate myelin production. One of the biggest factors of neurological damage at the change of life is that the hypothalamus no longer produces adequate amounts of GnRH. Not only does GnRH stimulate reproduction and sex hormone production, but it stimulates nerve rejuvenation. The worsening of symptoms that we see in multiple sclerosis patients at the change of life may be attributed to disturbances in the hypothalamic-pituitary-gonadal axis, including a diminishing production of GnRH.

By providing bio-identical hormone replacement therapy, we can help to correct some of the hypothalamic-pituitary-gonadal miscommunication and also utilize the growth factors that sex hormones provide to stimulate nerve rejuvenation and myelin sheath production. Progesterone is particularly effective at stimulating myelin sheath growth.

Unfortunately, it is uncommon for healthcare providers to provide progesterone with testosterone replacement therapy for men in andropause, since progesterone is believed to be a female hormone. Yet, both sexes produce progesterone, mainly by the adrenals in males. By midlife, the adrenals function at a lower level.

Progesterone is a natural aromatase inhibitor, so when initiating testosterone replacement therapy without progesterone, there is more conversion to estradiol which can increase body fat composition in men.

In andropausal men, we need to maintain adequate androgen levels to improve their symptoms and increase bone and muscle mass. For Richard, he needs enough testosterone and progesterone to help with nerve rejuvenation and myelin sheath repair. We're also going to introduce some specific nutraceuticals that can help with myelin sheath repair.

My favorite is CDP choline. Cytidine 5'-diphosphocholine (CDP-choline or citicoline) is an essential intermediate in the biosynthetic pathway of the structural phospholipids of cell membranes. Research on CDP choline shows its effectiveness in traumatic brain injury and dementia. Its main use is to help re-myelinate damaged neurons.

Yet, trying to repair damage while the immune system is actively attacking the central nervous system is like trying to build a sand castle too close to the waves. We must focus on calming down the hyper-immune response. In Richard's case, we also want to investigate potential heavy metal toxicity that may be stimulating his autoimmunity. So, we conduct a provoked urine toxicology.

Heavy Metal Toxicity and Autoimmunity

Research indicates that metals have the potential to induce or promote the development of autoimmunity. Metal-induced inflammation may dysregulate the hypothalamic-pituitary-adrenal (HPA) axis and thus, contribute to fatigue and other non-specific symptoms characterizing disorders related to autoimmune diseases. The toxic effects of several metals are also mediated through free radical formation, cell membrane disturbance and enzyme inhibition.

The kidneys pull out toxins from the bloodstream including heavy metals that may be leaching from the bones, brain, liver and other glandular tissues. Since Richard's exposure was more than 40 years ago, we need to do a provocation test. Typically, provocation tests use a well-known chelator

- dimercapto succinic acid (DMSA) - to pull heavy metals stored deeply in the tissues. We're not going to pull all the heavy metals in just one diagnostic provocation, but we will get an idea of what Richard's body has been storing.

Provoked urine toxicology is the gold standard test. Blood analysis reveals acute ingestion of heavy metals. When Richard was in puberty being exposed to arsenic that would have been the time to check his blood levels, similar to checking blood levels of lead paint exposure in young children. Hair analysis shows what has been leaching out into the bloodstream over the past six to eight weeks. We need to go deeper.

DMSA is like a magnet drawing heavy metals out of tissues. If it draws more than it can hold, the heavy metals may be reabsorbed by the central nervous system. An excellent protector of the central nervous system is alpha lipoic acid (ALA). A provoked urine toxicology is best done over three days taking DMSA with ALA three times a day. If patients experience headaches during the chelation, they're going to need to use ALA for a couple of days before and after each chelation. Urine is collected for 24 hours from day three to four. Then a specimen of the 24 hour urine collection is sent out to a lab to evaluate for heavy metals.

Richard's provoked urine toxicology reveals high levels of arsenic as well as a little mercury, lead and barium most likely from some former radiological testing. We start chelation therapy to pull out the arsenic and other heavy metals with both DMSA and ALA for three days every two weeks. After the eighth chelation we'll retest. Removing excess heavy metal burden can help calm down his autoimmune response contributing to MS.

Richard's blood results reveal:

- Slightly elevated PSA, with high free PSA, indicating benign prostatic hypertrophy. Low levels of free PSA with high PSA are an ominous sign.

- Testosterone is low at 220 supporting the assessment of andropause.

- ANA is elevated indicating continued autoimmune cell destruction.

- Liver function tests reveal elevated enzymes, both AST and ALT, which is not surprising with his long term drug abuse.

The T · P factor

While andropause happens to all men, over the past few decades, men have become more estrogenized with lower testosterone at younger ages. Hypogonadism or abnormally low androgen production is due to poor diet, especially eating too many carbohydrates. Men with insulin resistance convert more of their testosterone into estrogen. Plus exposure to xenoestrogens in the environment is reducing male testosterone. Hypogonadism is also due to inactivity, not exercising as much as the male body needs. Being sedentary is like smoking. It'll eventually shorten your life.

I prescribe compounded transdermal testosterone for Richard. I always have men apply it on their upper inner arms because studies show it's the best place for testosterone absorption. I also put a tiny bit of progesterone in with testosterone.

Progesterone is a natural aromatase inhibitor. Blocking this enzyme will help to prevent conversion of testosterone into estrogen. Excess dihydrotestosterone (DHT) will cause further enlargement of his prostate. So, we will block his DHT at cell receptor sites using saw palmetto.

If Richard had a menstruating partner, he would take a break from his hormones for three days when she has her period. If she's menopausal and on BHRT, they would take their three day breaks together. Why? Because studies show that men's hormones follow their female partners.

I will not prescribe testosterone if Richard is not going to be able to exercise because testosterone will stimulate growth of abnormal tissue. Testosterone is anabolic meaning growth promoting, just like estrogen is a growth factor for women.

All of my hormonally challenged patients must follow up with me so I can help them adjust their hormones. Once they learn what the hormones are doing and how to make the adjustments, we can meet annually, but in the first year it's once a month for three months, then every three months to keep them in balance.

Covid and Hypothalamus Dysfunction

When Covid shut us down in March 2020, I joined an online group of Covid survivors to see what they were describing. I suspected, like EBV, SARS-COV-19 was going to have similar effects on the body long-term. The survivors suffered from severe fatigue, brain fog, depression, POTS, new onset hormone issues, menstrual irregularities, erectile dysfunction, hair loss, etc. - symptoms highly suggestive of hypothalamic dysfunction. And about two months after I joined the group, French researchers found that the hypothalamus was being affected by Covid because it's rich in ACE2 receptors.

The hypothalamus is not protected by the blood brain barrier. So what other infections and toxins may be damaging the hypothalamus? Because the hypothalamus is orchestrating every vital system - your neurological system, your immune system, your endocrine system, detoxification, digestion and metabolism - it's important that we pay attention to hypothalamic insults like SARS-COV-19.

In the next two decades, we will see an increase in metabolic conditions like diabetes which will lead to early onset cardiovascular disease, disability and death all from so many people being infected with Covid. Mitigating the effects of long Covid is yet another reason hypothalamus support is foundational to long-term health and well-being.

While Richard's chief complaint is long Covid symptoms, his case is complicated by MS, andropause and addiction.

Dealing with Addiction

Millions of people from all walks of life struggle with addiction to drugs and alcohol. Research has shown that stress exposures – especially in early life – enhance illicit drug use and are the precipitating factors to many relapses in people with addiction. There are notable changes in the hypothalamic-pituitary-adrenal axis and hypothalamic autonomic arousal in addicted people.

The pathophysiology of addiction revolves around the concepts of synaptic plasticity. Synaptic plasticity means the ability of the brain to change and adapt to new information. Long-term potentiation (LTP) is the phenomenon of strengthened neural connections overtime and with increased stimuli. LTP is how learning, habits and addictions get set in the brain. Long-term depression (LTD) is the decrease in the responsiveness of a neural signal with stimulation. LTD is the reason addicts need more and more drugs to get the same effect.

Many illicit substances interfere with sex hormone production. Opioids in particular affect GnRH production and cause oxidative stress at the cellular level further inhibiting nerve rejuvenation. Unfortunately, Richard's opiate addiction is still active which is going to make it a little harder to see the true effects of instituting bio-identical hormone replacement therapy. So, I have a frank discussion with Richard about his addictive behaviors. Opiates suppress the central nervous system. One thing that Richard doesn't need is suppression of his CNS. He will be more fatigued, have more brain fog and the CNS depression will interfere with his ability to rejuvenate his nerves.

Research has implicated dopamine as a pivotal neurotransmitter in the brain of an addict. Large and fast increases of dopamine have been associated with the onset and maintenance of addiction. As the addiction becomes chronic,

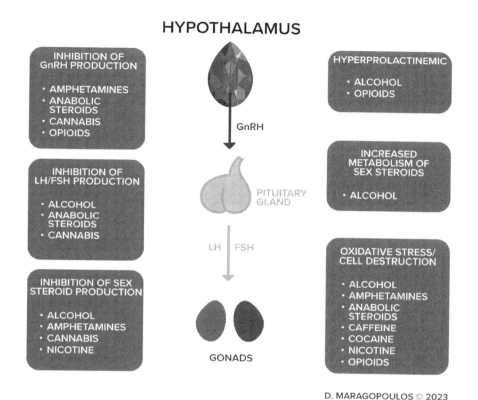

HYPOTHALAMUS

INHIBITION OF GnRH PRODUCTION

· AMPHETAMINES
· ANABOLIC STEROIDS
· CANNABIS
· OPIOIDS

INHIBITION OF LH/FSH PRODUCTION

· ALCOHOL
· ANABOLIC STEROIDS
· CANNABIS

INHIBITION OF SEX STEROID PRODUCTION

· ALCOHOL
· AMPHETAMINES
· CANNABIS
· NICOTINE

GnRH

PITUITARY GLAND

LH | FSH

GONADS

HYPERPROLACTINEMIC

· ALCOHOL
· OPIOIDS

INCREASED METABOLISM OF SEX STEROIDS

· ALCOHOL

OXIDATIVE STRESS/ CELL DESTRUCTION

· ALCOHOL
· AMPHETAMINES
· ANABOLIC STEROIDS
· CAFFEINE
· COCAINE
· NICOTINE
· OPIOIDS

D. MARAGOPOULOS © 2023

dopamine actually decreases, which is why supporting healthy hypothalamic dopamine production is essential to helping addicts live a sober life.

If you're making your own natural dopamine, you're less likely to give into addictive type behavior. So, I recommend adding extra Sacred Seven® hypothalamic amino acids to Richard's Genesis Gold®. The extra hypothalamic amino acids will increase dopamine production faster than Genesis Gold® alone.

Richard has not explored his childhood trauma in relation to why he started abusing substances in the first place. So, I recommend psychological therapy for Richard and after he's been evaluated, perhaps doing EMDR, to help him reset neurologically primed behaviors and try to break his addiction pattern.

According to his self-report, he's "just using hydrocodone as needed" as prescribed by a physician. Addicts have a tendency to underestimate how much they use, so we assume he's using more than the average person would use on a needed basis. Now, it's not going to be easy withdrawing from opiates. Withdrawal symptoms include severe gastrointestinal symptoms - pain, cramping and diarrhea. An over the counter medication - loperamide - can help with withdrawal. That's because loperamide fills opiate receptors in the gut. Unfortunately, many opiate addicts use excessive doses of loperamide and then become dependent on it. In small 2mg doses, up to eight milligrams per day, loperamide can be very helpful.

Richard is also committed to work with an addiction specialist who will evaluate him to see if he needs to be in an inpatient rehab. And to work on some of his deeper issues, especially since he hasn't really dealt with his adverse childhood experiences. Hopefully, the therapist will help him develop better coping mechanisms than using substances.

My assessment of Richard is hypothalamus dysfunction with multiple sclerosis, heavy metal toxicity, substance abuse disorder, and post-acute sequelae of SARS-Cov-2 infection.

Since Richard has had an autoimmune disorder for at least two decades with childhood heavy metal exposure and has been abusing substances for much longer, we will need to support optimal hypothalamus function for at least four years, although I suspect he will notice improvement in his symptoms within the first six to twelve months.

Here's what Richard's healing plan looks like:

1. Hypothalamus support - Genesis Gold® 4gm per 50 pounds of body weight with extra Sacred Seven® hypothalamic amino acids 5gm daily, mixed in water and taken every morning. Nutraceutical hypothalamus support will help Richard make more dopamine to begin overcoming his addiction, help suppress the autoimmune attack on his neurological system, improve his brain function, metabolism and energy and help him metabolize BHRT more safely.

2. Nutrition - Richard is going to start with a liver cleanse diet for seven days to help lower his liver enzymes. Then he'll proceed with my DMAR® Path to Nutritional Wellness. He has to pay attention to getting enough fatty acids especially omega-3s for their anti-inflammatory effect. Monounsaturated fatty acids from olive oil and avocado are essential to rebuild the myelin sheath. Plus, he needs to get phytonutrients from a variety of colorful vegetables, fruits, whole grains and legumes. He needs to make sure he's getting an adequate amount of protein to try to rebuild muscle tissue. With 140 pounds of lean body mass, he needs at least 100 grams of protein a day, 140 grams of protein would be better.

3. Activity - Exercise is essential to maintaining mobility and decreasing the disability that comes with multiple sclerosis. Whatever Richard can do, we're going to encourage him to do daily - both aerobic activity and weight resistance. I prescribe physical therapy to help work on muscle strength and coordination to help him with his balance and prevent falls.

4. Sleep - I recommend that Richard goes to bed at a reasonable time within three to four hours of dusk, so that he can get a deep enough sleep to benefit from nocturnal growth hormone production and help rejuvenate his myelin sheaths.

5. Mindset - Richard has been struggling with chronic illness and addiction most of his life with a mindset of defeat and victimhood. Helping him adopt a healing mindset will take therapy and time. I refer him to a therapist specializing in addictions. I counsel him on the use of creating structure in his life which will help control his stress reaction that triggers addictive behaviors.

6. CDP choline - To begin repairing myelin of his damaged nervous system. I recommend 2000mg daily for eight weeks, then 1000mg daily for four months then 500mg daily while MS is active.

7. Heavy metal chelation - DMSA 500mg and Alpha Lipoic Acid 400mg three times a day for three days every two weeks. On the eighth chelation, we will retest urine toxicology.

8. BHRT - Compounded transdermal cream containing testosterone 80mg plus 5mg of progesterone, applied to inner upper arms to help improve myelin sheath repair as well as improve sleep, mood and help him handle detoxification better. He's to take a break from BHRT at least three days per month.

Results

Richard reports improvement in his sleep, energy and brain fog within the first six weeks. He notices that if he forgets to take Genesis Gold® and Sacred Seven® that he definitely has more mental and physical fatigue.

In month two, Richard begins opiate withdrawal and loperamide 2mg up to four times daily for GI symptoms. It takes him three weeks to detox and another week to wean off loperamide.

By six months, Richard is happy to report that he's able to work as a contractor, able to keep up with the physical and mental stress of the job.

It takes Richard over a year to chelate arsenic and with consistent use of CDP choline, hormone replacement therapy and hypothalamic support, he notices a significant change in his MS symptoms.

Richard continues to support his hypothalamus, exercise, nourish his body and for the first time, he's maintained his sobriety. He's also learned some great stress reduction techniques that he's utilizing on a daily basis.

Chapter 8

Gender, Sexuality and Your Hypothalamus

One beautiful sunny summer afternoon, a nineteen year old patient who I've seen since they were three comes in for an annual physical. They are accompanied by their mother and girlfriend to discuss gender affirming care.

My patient is dressed in cargo pants, boots and a loose button up shirt. Their hair is cut short. Most noticeable is their cheerful demeanor. Since a very young age, my patient has been melancholy.

"You can call me Joseph."

From that moment on, his former name was put to rest for me and my staff.

A young transgender man, Joseph had been transitioning socially the past year. Now, he's asking for help with hormonal transition.

At Joseph's age, he's well past puberty so we need to introduce androgens to induce secondary male sexual characteristics. But first, I evaluate Joseph thoroughly. My concern for him is for his psychological and physical well-being.

Joseph was assigned female at birth, yet had always been uncomfortable in their body, depressed, ashamed of their form. My patient has struggled with depression, insulin resistance, and gastrointestinal issues.

As a female, my patient was not able to follow recommended diets or exercise to overcome their insulin resistance. They were depressed and never felt accepted by their extended family or friends.

As a transitioning male, my patient already appears happier. Still I want to be sure that the androgen therapy will not create metabolic issues.

So, following current protocol, I make sure that Joseph receives psychological counseling. Before starting gender affirming hormone therapy, it's very important that the patient is psychologically prepared for the changes.

Joseph has already started the social aspects of gender affirmation. While their immediate family is on board with their decision and very supportive, their extended family is not.

After a thorough evaluation, the psychotherapist who's well versed in transgender psychology, determines that Joseph would benefit psychologically and emotionally by receiving the hormones that matched their gender identity.

Of course, I start with a full endocrine panel to make sure everything else is functioning normally. Joseph comes to me with hyperprolactinemia which he has been dealing with for a while and not been able to correct without using a dopamine agonist. Joseph also has insulin resistance with an elevated HGBA1C though they're not overweight.

Whether transitioning male to female or female to male, we still want to look at the whole picture with a full endocrine panel. I want to check thyroid, adrenal glands and pituitary hormones. I'm going to check existing sex steroids along with pituitary FSH and LH, so I can get baselines. I want to look for signs of insulin resistance with hemoglobinA1C and C peptide levels.

I'm going to do a full examination of the patient to be sure that there are no other health issues and to evaluate their secondary sex characteristics, meaning facial hair, body hair, pubic line, breast development, body fat distribution, muscle tone and bone density before initiating therapy.

On physical examination, Joseph is endomorphic, with a congenital abdominal diastasis, and some acne on his cheeks and chin. Otherwise, his pre-transition exam is normal phenotypic female with slight bone structure and muscle mass, minimal body fat predominantly on hips and thighs, tanner stage 5 indicating postpubescent breast and pubic hair development. Tanner stages are guidelines for secondary sexual characteristic development and are rated from 0-6.

As per their usual behavior during physical examinations, my patient is quite self-conscious.

I explain during the examination what Joseph can expect from gender affirming hormone therapy - increase spread of pubic hair across groin and thighs as well as a linea towards his umbilicus, increase in acne extending onto neck, chest and back, facial hair growth, increase in musculature notably in arms, chest and back, thickening of neck and lowering of the voice as vocal cords thicken.

Joseph welcomes all these changes. "I can't wait. Will I feel better too?"

I hope so.

As healthcare providers, we want to make sure that we are contributing to our patients' health, vitality, longevity and happiness.

And counseling is not just for the patients undergoing transition. Counseling is also necessary for those who are dealing with the change in their family member.

This was not my first transgender patient.

In the early 90's, I was working in a private obgyn practice, taking care of a brand new patient who wanted to get her hormones refilled. Unfortunately, this patient did not feel comfortable providing their full history, stating that she had had a hysterectomy.

When I went in to examine her, it was obvious in my clinical assessment that this patient was a transwoman. Unfortunately, she had been exposed to so much prejudice in the medical field that she did not feel comfortable being candid with me. So, my job was to make her as comfortable as possible, give her the hormones that she needed and perform a gynecological exam. I also recommended a rectal Pap smear which at that time wasn't a very popular diagnostic test, but because of her sexual history, pre-transitioning, she was at risk for rectal HPV and carcinoma. Rectal Pap smears are an excellent diagnostic tool for both at risk males and females.

This lovely person was my initiation into the politics and controversy of the transgender world. Over the years, medical descriptions have changed. For instance, being transgender or transsexual used to be considered to be a psychiatric diagnosis.

Still, the medical society has definitely been slower in adopting change than the transgender community has needed. Even when an infant presents with ambiguous genitalia at birth, the medical community still advises that the parents choose a gender so the sex of the baby can be assigned. In our modern day society even with changing sexual roles, we are still defined by our genitalia.

Yet, how can black and white definitions of male and female reflect the effects of hormones on the brain, specifically identity and emotional development? While there are clear differences between the infant male and female brain, studies show that gay men have brain development and activity more like ciswomen than cismen.

As the mother of an infant born with ambiguous genitalia, I was told to choose a side - male or female. My infant had XY chromosomes, yet appeared female in their genitalia development. Female is the default in fetal development. Unless there's enough testosterone and functioning receptors to receive testosterone, fetal genital development will appear female or ambiguous.

It was 1984 and the top pediatric endocrinologist in California labeled our baby an XY female. The term intersex was not been coined until the early 90s'. In spite of my infants' male chromosomes, the endocrinologist said it was "easier to make a hole than a pole" so it was best to raise our child as a female and later perform sex reassignment surgery. I did not agree.

As of the writing of this book, parents are still only given two choices at birth - male or female. Although now, parents are steered towards following the infant's chromosomes, not necessarily their genital appearance.

I went against standard accepted medical advice and had to navigate the very complex medical system alone to try to get my intersex child the care that they needed.

It's not easy raising a child who is unhappy in their body. It's not easy navigating a medical system that does not recognize the child's psychological well-being, but only sees the child as a medical aberration and a potential experiment.

I have much empathy as a parent and healthcare provider for people navigating the system to get the care they need. And I'm very much empathetic to parents, children and adults who are dealing with trying to get gender affirming care.

Navigating Gender Identity

Are there just two genders? I don't believe so.

In indigenous cultures, there exists a third gender - a middle sex - where gender and sexuality are not black and white but more of a rainbow of possibility. Intersexuality - being born with ambiguous genitalia, receptor site issues, chromosome aberrations like extra Xs or Ys, hermaphroditism - is estimated to occur in 1-2 out of 100 births, as common as having red hair.

While it is difficult for people to change how they relate to family members who transition, imagine how difficult it is for the individual to feel one way and be treated by their family and society as something else?

Gender as a role is defined by societal norms. The profound shift in female roles over the last century is a prime example. Today's women are leaders, scientists, police officers, soldiers and astronauts. Women are no longer defined by who they're married to but have carved out their own identity. And men have learned to adapt, taking over some traditional female roles like childcare.

So, is gender defined by society or is it innate?

Let's look at the John/Joan case study.

In 1967, psychologist John Money encouraged the gender reassignment of David Reimer, who was born a biological male but suffered irreparable damage to his penis as an infant due to a failed circumcision. Money encouraged

Reimer's parents to raise him as a girl which they did, including surgery to remove his testes, create rudimentary female genitalia, and administering female hormones at puberty.

Reimer was an identical twin so the psychologist tracked the twins' development, hence, the John/Joan case study. Except Money reported erroneous results because Reimer clearly displayed gender dysphoria and by mid-teens identified as a male. Later, he underwent gender reassignment hormones and surgery, married a woman, but suffered severe depression and at the age of 38, committed suicide.

The John/Joan case provided results that were used to justify thousands of sex reassignment surgeries for cases of children with reproductive abnormalities. Except Money never reported how unhappy "Joan" was.

Like all parents of intersex children born in the 70s - 90's, due to the erroneous reports from this one twin study, my husband and I were guided to raise our child according to their genitalia not their chromosomes. Not until the late 90's did Reimer's public statements about the trauma of his transition bring attention to gender identity and called into question the sex assignment of infants and children.

Because we chose our child's chromosomes, not their genital appearance, our child used male pronouns for the first three decades of their life. While it's easy for me to refer to my firstborn as they/them when I'm writing or speaking, in a family situation, since we identified this child with male pronouns, it's been harder to consistently use non gendered pronouns. A year ago, we adopted a kitten with hermaphroditism (yes, intersex is just as common in the animal kingdom) which has helped us practice using they/them.

Not that I was surprised when my adult child identified as non-binary. From birth, they were fluid in their gender identity. While it's common for very young children to play both traditional male or female roles, my child continued to flow between male and female behaviors through their adolescence and into young adulthood.

We encouraged our child to be who they were, yet, we did have to decide when our child was just an infant whether to preserve their gonads. Our child was born with large inguinal hernias that prevented them from normal defecation. Having trained at UCLA, I worked with a urological surgeon who had performed some of the first transgender affirming surgeries. Our baby's hernias needed to be repaired, but their testes were in their abdomen and their ambiguous genitalia did not include a scrotum. If the testes are not removed or brought down and attached into the scrotum, they become cancerous. We decided not to remove their gonads.

Although our child had partial androgen insensitivity, I had a dream that giving our child testosterone would allow the surgeon to have enough tissue to bring the testes down. And it worked. Two decades later, testosterone challenge became the standard of care for children born with ambiguous genitalia and XY chromosomes.

As for our child's identity, we named them a very ambiguous name. The pediatric endocrinologist did not agree, advising the child be named a more traditional masculine name. Our concern was that this child may not be happy with our choice of gender assignment. So, we chose a name for our child that they could keep for the rest of their life in case we were premature in assuming how they wanted to identify themselves.

Another issue the endocrinologist had was with our non gender style of parenting. Our child was very interested in playing house and especially in cooking, so my husband made them a play kitchen. The physician believed cooking to be a female role. However, my Greek husband is a very good cook and spends lots of time in the kitchen. Working shift work, we shared childcare, so our firstborn emulated both of us. Today, we wouldn't think anything of it, both little boys and little girls play in the kitchen. Times have changed a lot in terms of how we look at gender roles.

By the time our child was in early elementary school, they loved super heros and played with toys like weapons. Even though my husband was a police officer, we discouraged gun play since our two year old nephew accidentally shot himself. Still, our firstborn would pretend to shoot with sticks and bananas. Throughout elementary school, their playmates went from female to male. By high school, they were involved in drama and chorus and had a mixed group of friends.

Our child went to college in San Francisco which ended up being a very good place for them to be because they were able to get the help they needed with their gender dysphoria. They joined a transgender queer therapy group, but found that it really didn't address the issues of intersex people. So with the help of a licensed therapist, they started an intersex group.

Let me explain intersexuality on a spectrum. There's not clearly male and female in humans or the animal kingdom. There are variations of masculine and feminine. There are variations not just in expression, but in genetics. We see variations of sex chromosome combinations that result in different physical expressions, so different genitalia, different secondary sex characteristics, as well as psychological and social expression.

Perhaps, it's a journey for people with gender dysphoria, being defined by society and not in sync with how they feel, how their brain functions and how their body looks and feels.

I am a cis-female clinician - mother to a cis-female daughter and an intersex child. My pronouns are she/her. My granddaughter has been exposed to all genders and fluidly uses non-binary pronouns for non-binary people.

The question of whether gender is defined by nature or nurture is still unanswered. In the meantime, I will continue to provide the most conscious compassionate care I can for all my patients no matter how they identify.

Do hormones affect physiology?

Absolutely! And my transgender patient, Joseph, is a fine example of how hormones affect physiology. Studies have shown that hormones affect longevity too. Cis-females and transmen live longer than cis-males, while transwomen have the shortest lifespan. It appears that being born biologically female increases longevity no matter what hormones you're exposed to. Longevity studies in transgender people are skewed as there's a high rate of accidental death due to homocide and suicide in trans-youth bringing the average age of longevity down considerably compared to cis-people.

We know hormones affect brain function but let's look at something we all share no matter what gender we identify with - our guts. Studies show that gut function is influenced by hormones too. The hypothalamus coordinates gastrointestinal activity and communicates directly with the microbiome of the gut.

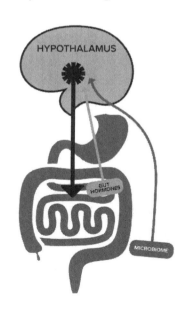

My patient had always had gut issues. I always suspected that she had an intestinal imbalance, but once we transitioned her to him, he did not. As a child, my patient had abnormal digestion, poor nutrient absorption and chronic intestinal dysbiosis - which means the gut microbiome was out of balance. My patient would get bloated after eating, sometimes constipated, and when stressed would suffer from diarrhea.

How can we look at the gut? By evaluating a stool specimen, we can determine gut function including microbiome health. We can check digestive markers like pH and determine pancreatic enzyme and bile activity by checking protein and fat absorption. Through stool analysis, we can check for pathogenic microbes including bacteria, fungus and parasites. We can measure inflammatory markers that may indicate infection, allergy, innate gut immunity, and membrane permeability. Most importantly, through stool analysis, we can determine beneficial microbiome numbers, diversity and activity.

Just like a stress treadmill is a more accurate evaluation than an EKG to determine cardiac function, a functional stool analysis gives us more information than a simple stool culture and sensitivity or parasitology.

Even endoscopic evaluations do not provide this same information about gut function and microbiome health. Today, we can do fecal DNA evaluations to help determine colon cancer. Of course, if we suspect cancer, a referral to a gastroenterologist for colonoscopy or endoscopy is indicated. The gastroenterologist can see tumors, polyps, ulcers, even signs of gastritis but they can't see gut function. A functional stool analysis gives us the information we need about intestinal function including digestion, absorption and microbiome health.

Let's follow the path of digestion and see what might go wrong.

Digestion starts in the mouth. Saliva is rich in amylase which breaks down to simple carbohydrates. Sugar can be absorbed right though the large vessel under the tongue. Food is then masticated (chewed) before going down the esophagus through the pyloric sphincter and into the stomach. Gastric juices are supposed to be very acidic with a pH of one. In comparison, water is neutral with a pH of seven. Thankfully, the stomach makes mucus to protect it from gastric acid, otherwise it would digest itself.

Masticated food broken down by highly acidic stomach acid is called chyme. When chyme is passed through the duodenal sphincter and into the small intestine, whatever's at the end of the small intestine is dumped through the ileocecal valve into the large intestine.

Gastrointestinal hormones play a role in proper digestion and absorption. As soon as the duodenal valve at the bottom of the stomach opens up, a hormone called cholecystokinin (CCK) is secreted by cells in the duodenum and stimulates the release of bile into the intestine and the secretion of enzymes by the pancreas.

The hormone secretin stimulates biliary and pancreatic ductular cells to secrete bicarbonate and water in response to the presence of acid in the duodenum to expand the volume of bile entering the duodenum.

Bile helps to promote lipid absorption as the conjugated bile acids emulsify lipids while escorting them through the jejunum into the distal small intestine - the ileum - for efficient absorption into the mesentery arteries. The web of mesentery arteries carry nutrients and bile acids through the hepatic portal to the liver. Conjugated bile acids are recycled one or more times with each meal. Bile also carries waste products, bilirubin and cholesterol to be eliminated through the feces.

Bile is a pH of nine so it effectively neutralizes acidic stomach chime, thereby preventing a duodenal ulcer. Plus, pancreatic enzymes can only function at a pH of 6.8 - 7.2. If you don't have a gallbladder, bile will be dumped directly from the liver bile ducts into the duodenum.

Bile acts as an antimicrobial to protect the small intestine. The production of bile requires amino acids taurine and glycine, cholesterol, vitamin C, and lecithin. Vitamin C is needed for the enzymatic conversion of cholesterol to bile salts. Taurine and glycine are conjugated with bile salts. Phosphatidylcholine is crucial for bile flow support by preventing sludgy bile.

Bile acids emulsify fats so that pancreatic lipase enzymes can break down fat into long chain fatty acids and beneficial bacteria break down fat into short chain fatty acids to be absorbed in the small intestine. Proteases break down proteins and amylases break down carbohydrates. Compared to the large intestine the small intestine is very long, about 24 feet, with lots of surface area for absorption of nutrients. Micronutrients like amino acids, fatty acids, vitamins and minerals as well as macronutrients like carbohydrates, proteins and fats are absorbed through the permeable membrane of the small intestine and into the bloodstream.

From there, nutrients as well as toxins pass through the liver. The liver is the body's filter to catch toxins before they're released into the bloodstream. The undigested waste then passes through the ileocecal valve and into the large intestine (colon). The colon is only eight feet long but a very large diameter compared to the small intestine. The colon cells are spaced just far enough apart to create a transpermeable membrane which is designed to allow water in and out of the colon to help form a passable stool. Too much water in the colon causes diarrhea. Too little water causes constipation. If the colon epithelial cells are damaged, food particles and toxins pass through and into the bloodstream. When a damaged colon lining allows more than water to get through and into the bloodstream, often called a leaky gut, the immune system reacts violently which can result in allergies and autoimmunity.

Prior to transitioning, Joseph's stool analysis indicated candida overgrowth and poor digestion of proteins and fats. They craved carbohydrates which elevated their blood glucose levels. They also tended to get bloated after eating and so experienced flatulence (gas).

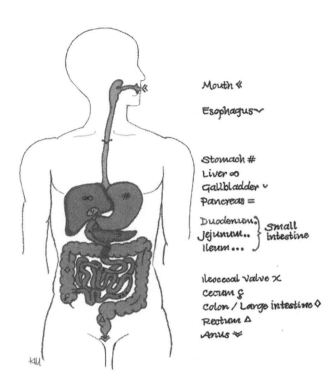

Mouth «

Esophagus ⌄

Stomach #
Liver ∞
Gallbladder ⌄
Pancreas =

Duodenum. ⎫
Jejunum.. ⎬ Small
Ileum ... ⎭ intestine

Ileocecal Valve X
Cecum ʃ
Colon / Large intestine ◊
Rectum △
Anus ⩔

The odor of gas sometimes indicates which microbe is the most active. Particularly, foul gas can indicate bacterial overgrowth and can be induced by any food. The most foul gas may indicate infection with Giardia. An overgrowth of candida causes excess bloating and gas after consuming starchy carbohydrates.

With a stool analysis, a culture and sensitivity can be performed, meaning the pathogens are grown in a Petri dish, then tested for their sensitivity to antimicrobial discs impregnated with antibiotics, antifungals or antimicrobial botanicals. Unlike resistant pathogens which grow right over the antimicrobial, if the pathogens are sensitive to the antimicrobial there's no growth around the disc. I prefer to prescribe the antimicrobial that the offending agent is most sensitive to - natural or chemical. Botanical antimicrobials like oregano oil and berberine can be useful in eradicating intestinal dysbiosis.

After being exposed to androgens, Joseph's stool analysis corrected itself. He craved more protein foods and less starchy carbs helping to reduce his HGBA1C. I counseled him to go slowly in introducing more protein. Initially, he had some issues with maldigestion as his stomach acid and bile production needed to increase from his previous carb rich diet to digest a more protein based diet. Joseph's increased hunger led to more frequent feedings and he began to complain of gas and bloating after eating, which may indicate SIBO or small intestinal bacterial overgrowth.

Sometimes, the ileocecal valve allows bacteria from the colon up into the small intestines. This displaced bacteria causes fermentation of partially digested food leading to gas and bloating. For proper digestion and to prevent ileocecal valve leakage, it's best to space meals at least four hours apart. SIBO is diagnosed by a breath test after the patient drinks glucose. An overgrowth of bacteria in the small intestine causes an elevation in methane and/or hydrogen gases.

Joseph's breath test showed an elevation in hydrogen gas which is best treated by the non-systemic antibiotic rifampin. SIBO can be difficult to eradicate, so rifampin can be followed by a course of berberine and oregano oil. Repeat testing may need to be done if the patient remains symptomatic. Increasing bile flow can help to protect the small intestine from bacterial overgrowth. Allowing the liver to produce enough bile by fasting from dusk to dawn and consuming bitters like lemon water with meals can help to increase bile flow. Spacing meals at least four hours apart helps to prevent ileocecal reflux of colon bacteria into the small intestine.

My assessment of Joseph is hypothalamus dysfunction with gender dysphoria, intestinal dysbiosis, insulin resistance, and hyperprolactinemia.

Since Joseph is just beginning gender affirming hormones, we will need to support optimal hypothalamus function for at least two years, although I suspect resolution of his metabolic issues within the first year.

Here's what Joseph's healing plan looks like:

1. Hypothalamus support - Genesis Gold® 4gm per 50 pounds of body weight mixed in water and taken frost thing in the morning. Nutraceutical hypothalamus support will help Joseph metabolize androgens more safely and support adequate receptor function. Continued hypothalamus support will help maintain metabolic health as well as decrease potential hypothalamic microinflammation as he transitions.

2. Nutrition - I recommend DMAR® Path to Nutritional Wellness. Joseph needs to make sure he's getting an adequate amount of protein to try to build muscle tissue. With 90 pounds of lean body mass, he needs at least 75 grams of protein a day increasing to 150 grams daily to maintain a more masculine physique. Joseph also needs to be sure he's getting enough phytonutrients from a variety of colorful vegetables, fruits, whole grains, legumes to help him metabolize androgens safely.

3. Activity - Weight resistance exercise is critical to building muscle mass under the influence of androgens. For his cardiovascular health, I recommend 30 minutes of aerobic activity at least three times a week.

4. Sleep - Joseph has always been a good sleeper. So, we continue to support good sleep hygiene with limited screen time after dusk and sleeping in a cool dark room. I recommend Joseph get up with the sun to help increase serotonin production.

5. Mindset - Once Joseph received gender affirming care, his mindset shifted. He looked at the world in a more positive way and felt more comfortable in his body. I recommend continuing to receive psychological counseling throughout his transition period.

6. Gender affirming care - Testosterone 80mg + progesterone 5mg in liposomal transdermal cream to be applied to upper inner arms twice daily for three months, then take a 3 day break every three months. Recheck testosterone, dihydrotestosterone, estradiol and SHBG levels at one month, three months, six months, then yearly.

7. To eradicate SIBO - I advise Joseph to space his meals at least four hours apart and prescribe Rifampin 550mg three times daily for 14 days. If symptoms recur, we'll recheck breath test and if positive, start antimicrobial botanicals - berberine 500mg twice daily and oregano oil capsules 300 mg twice daily for three weeks. I advise that Joseph drink lemon water with each meal to stimulate bile flow and include bitter greens, dandelion, milk thistle, berries, and beetroot in his diet.

Results

Once we start gender affirming hormone therapy, what I observe in my patient is short of a miracle. This depressed young person became motivated to take care of themselves.

Joseph began sleeping better and started exercising regularly. Most importantly, Joseph was enjoying the changes that they were noticing in their body which at first was facial hair growth and increased musculature.

My patient was finally happy.

And his metabolic issues resolved. Within a couple of months, his elevated HGBA1C lowered and finally his prolactin decreased to acceptable daytime levels.

A couple years into providing gender affirming hormones and after extensive counseling, Joseph was ready to undergo bilateral mastectomy.

While his estrogen levels in the female range contributed to hyperprolactinemia, insulin resistance and depression, testosterone reversed everything for Joseph. Yet, testosterone is not known to reverse insulin resistance or depression or hyperprolactinemia.

Which made me wonder what's happening in the brain, specifically the hypothalamus, during fetal development that attunes it to certain sex steroids.

What are the biological adaptations to available hormones and how does it affect our brain development and sense of self?

More studies will need to be done to answer these questions. In the meantime, I will be treating my patients with personalized protocols based on empirical data. And continue to encourage my patients to support their hypothalamus nutraceutically to help with their transition and beyond.

As a family nurse practitioner, I am very much aware that we need to pay attention to the general health of transgender people so that they can get all the care they need. Personalized holistic healthcare that pays attention to how gender affirming hormones affects their physical metabolism and mental health is vital. We want to make sure that the hormones that we're giving our transgender patients are helping, not causing, metabolic issues.

To witness Joseph's transformation from metabolic inflammation to health, and more so happiness, confirmed in my mind that sex hormones affect way more than reproduction and sexuality.

I have known this child since they were three and helped them transition sixteen years later. Even though they've only been living their life as a male for just a few years, when I first started writing this piece, I couldn't remember their birth name. I only remember them as who they are now.

Perhaps that's because who they are now is who they were meant to be. And as a clinician, it makes me very happy to see that my patient's health is no longer compromised. The gender affirming hormones seemed to correct more than their psychological well-being; it corrected their innate metabolism.

Chapter 9

Developmental Delay, Learning and Your Hypothalamus

On an overcast winter morning, three-year-old Christina comes in with her parents and five-year-old brother. Christina is showing signs of developmental delay and in spite of seeing multiple providers, her parents are unable to get a working diagnosis. They're also interested in more natural approaches for Christina's health and well-being.

I sit down on the floor to observe my new patient. At 38 months, Christina engages with me in play. She laughs when I use a puppet to talk to her but does not respond verbally. She brings me the toys I ask for but does not seem to know her colors or shapes. I note that she had trouble stacking blocks.

Her gait is wide stanced. She tries to mimic me in touching her knees and shoulders. She can jump up and down but has trouble balancing on one foot.

Christina points and gestures when she wants something. She not only looks me in the eye but picks up a book and climbs into my lap. We end our play assessment with coloring. Christina has trouble holding a slender crayon and uses her fist to hold a thick crayon. She can not draw any shapes I request, nor copy mine.

She walked late at 17 months and her gross motor skills are behind at the age of three. Her fine motor skills are markedly behind. My developmental assessment of Christina puts her at 18-20 months with aphasia.

Christina's mother reports that her pregnancy was uneventful. She was in fairly good health, before and during the pregnancy, but her delivery was fraught with issues. Christina was delivered at 41 weeks by induction. A week prior, Christina's mother noticed that the baby was not as active and went in to be checked by her midwife who sent her in for a non-stress test. The non-stress tests showed some fetal bradycardia and she was kept overnight to see if the baby had heart rate variability. After 24 hours of monitoring, she was released by her obstetrician back into her midwife's care.

Within a couple of days, Christina's mother started signs of labor. After five days of inactive labor, Christina's mother went back to the labor and delivery unit to be induced. Induction did not last long as Christina's heart rate dropped considerably and she had to be delivered via emergency C-section.

Christina's apgars were low, so she spent time in the NICU with oxygen. Today, Christina would have put in a cooling blanket to lower her brain metabolism and hopefully prevent further brain damage. Thankfully, Christina did not develop infantile seizures.

Christina's parents were able to bring her home at five days of age. Her mother breastfed her for the first year of her life, followed by a fairly healthy diet of organic foods and tried to limit toxic exposures for both of her children.

Christina received recommended childhood immunizations and had normal early childhood upper respiratory infections, nothing of concern.

Her mother noticed in her first year that Christina wasn't developing as quickly as her older brother had and brought her concerns to the pediatrician. Her pediatrician did a developmental assessment on Christina at 12 months and at that point, she had just started crawling and was babbling but her development was definitely slow.

At 18 months, Christina suffered a head injury due to a fall and had a CT scan done which showed some hypoplasia of her pituitary. Her mother did not feel that her development was any more delayed after the head injury and wondered if this was Christina's baseline.

College educated, Christina's mother has done extensive research on how to help her. Christina's father owns a business in agriculture and does have toxic exposures to pesticides and herbicides. Christina's five-year-old brother has normal development for his age and engages well with his little sister. Christina has two dogs and a cat at home and is also exposed to farm animals as they live in the country. She is very happy when playing outside. She becomes emotionally distraught with abrupt changes in her schedule.

On her physical exam, I note that the tags had been removed from her clothing. Christina's mother confirms that she's sensitive to some textiles as well as loud noises.

Christina is of average height, weight and head circumference for her age. Her facial features are symmetrical. The rest of her physical exam is normal except a wide abdominal rectus diastasis. I show mother and child some exercises to help strengthen Christina's abdominal muscles which should help her balance and gross motor skill development.

Christina's mother is concerned that Christina may have sustained a brain injury at birth that wasn't detected. I suspect that Christina probably suffered hypoxic ischemic encephalopathy - in which her brain did not get enough oxygen shortly before or during her birth. In spite of her mother's effort to provide a healthy diet and environment, Christina didn't receive the early infant stimulation she needed for optimal brain development.

My goal with Christina is to provide her with enough support developmentally and nutritionally in order to help her be able to communicate her needs and learn at a more accelerated rate than she's currently able to. Although Christina does show some mild signs of autism spectrum disorder, it was not the diagnosis that she was given by child behavioral specialists when I first saw this child over twenty years ago. Her diagnosis was learning disabilities of unknown origin. Birth trauma, like hypoxic ischemic encephalopathy, does not show changes in the brain on early scans, but can show changes in the second year of life.

I suspect that Christina's head trauma, while a good opportunity to do a brain scan, may not have contributed to her underlying neurological condition. For this three-year-old, I order some basic blood panels - chemistry, CBC and because of her smaller than normal pituitary gland, prolactin, TSH and IGF-1 levels. All of Christina's labs are within normal limits.

Because of her father's work potentially exposing the family to toxins, I order a noninvasive hair analysis to test for heavy metal exposure. Christina has moderate levels of lead and mercury, confirmed on a provoked urine toxicology.

Our plan to help Christina is to provide hypothalamic and developmental support. Genesis Gold® can easily be mixed into water or juice, and for young children, applesauce or yogurt to provide her hypothalamus-pituitary axis with the nutrients it needs to prevent hypothalamic micro-inflammation. We're also going to be sure that this child gets an adequate amount of omega 3 rich polyunsaturated fats particularly DHA. I also recommend speech and occupational therapy to help Christina and teach her family how to best help her develop.

What is the hypothalamus' role in learning and development?

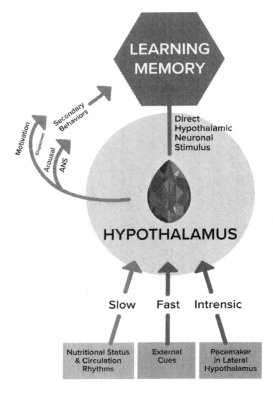

D. MARAGOPOULOS © 2023

The lateral aspect of the hypothalamus is involved in reward and reinforcement processes of learning, memory and behavioral control. The hypothalamus is the main producer of dopamine which enhances learning and memory through the reward pathways.

The lateral hypothalamic GABA neurons contribute to associative learning. Associative learning happens when two unrelated elements (objects, sights, sounds, ideas, and/or behaviors) become linked.

Children who are exposed to high stress environments including infants who are separated from their mothers at birth tend to develop hypersentive hypothalamic-pituitary-adrenal axis. Sustained activation of the HPA axis can lead to impairments in learning and memory. That's because adrenaline stimulates neuroexcitatory effects on the brain, while GABA calmly paces learning and sets memory.

Early life experiences govern the expression of stress related genes throughout life.

There is evidence that hypothalamic damage impacts memory retrieval which may be what we're seeing in long Covid and traumatic brain injuries including birth trauma.

It's vitally important that women in their reproductive years are hormonally balanced with optimal hypothalamic function as their health affects their developing fetus. For instance, thyroid hormone is essential for normal brain development and function, and the fetus is dependent on maternal thyroid hormone supply. Just before birth, the fetal hypothalamus stimulates an increase in thyrotropin (TSH) to begin neonatal thyroid hormone production.

The hypothalamus plays an important role in early neurobehavioral development through its involvement in the developing stress reaction of the preterm infant and its communication with the prefrontal cortex which is the locus of cognition and executive functions.

While the brains of autistic children are no different in size than control children, their hypothalamus is smaller. The hypothalamic hormones oxytocin and vasopressin have been documented to support and regulate socio-emotional responses. Both oxytocin and vasopressin are often poorly expressed in autistic children.

Human cognition is highly dependent on hypothalamus dopamine, neuro-trophins, and healthy gut microbiome.

Dopamine is involved in motor planning and higher order cognitive abilities - reasoning, language comprehension, future projection and general intelligence.

Neurotrophins are growth promoters of nerves and include brain derived neurotrophic factor (BDNF), vascular endothelial growth factor (VEGF) and insulin like growth factor (IGF). Studies show that hypothalamic dys-function affects neurotrophic production and activity.

The gut microbiome communicates directly with the hypothalamus and directs neuro-hormonal regulation. Compromised gut microbiome has recently been shown to contribute to many psychiatric and immunological disorders. Gut bacterial species also play an important role in neonatal brain development by modulating neurotrophins.

The gut bacteria takes approximately 2–3 years before it resembles the adult microbiome. Breastfeeding helps the baby's gut to colonize if the mother's gut microbiome is healthy and diversified.

While healthy mothers are more likely to have healthy babies, brain injuries at birth can contribute to developmental disabilities.

What are developmental disabilities?

Developmental disabilities are a group of conditions due to an impairment in physical, learning, language, or behavior. About one in six children in the U.S. have one or more developmental disabilities or other developmental delays.

A child is considered developmentally delayed if they have not gained the developmental skills expected of them, compared to children of the same age. Delays may occur in motor function, speech and language, cognitive, play and social skills.

Developmental disabilities are identified before the age of 22, and usually last throughout a person's lifetime. These disabilities include intellectual disabilities, cerebral palsy, autism spectrum disorder, Down syndrome, language and learning disorders, vision impairment, and hearing loss.

Developmental disabilities are differences that are usually present at birth and that uniquely affect the trajectory of the individual's physical, intellectual, and/or emotional development. Developmental disabilities may affect the ability to learn, reason, problem solve and other skills; as well as adaptive behavior, which includes everyday social and life skills.

Developmental disabilities may affect different body systems:

Nervous system disorders

Nervous system disorders affect how the brain, spinal cord and peripheral nervous system function, which can affect intelligence and learning. These conditions can also cause other issues, such as behavioral disorders, speech or language difficulties, seizures and trouble with movement. Cerebral palsy, Down syndrome, Fragile X syndrome and autism spectrum disorders (ASDs) are examples of intellectual and developmental disabilities caused by disorders of the nervous system.

Sensory system disorders

Sensory system disorders affect the senses (sight, hearing, touch, taste, and smell) or how the brain processes or interprets information from the senses. Preterm infants and infants exposed to infections, such as cytomegalovirus, may have reduced function with their eyesight and/or hearing. The sense of touch and sound can be hypersensitive in people with autism spectrum disorders.

Metabolic disorders

Metabolic disorders affect how the body uses food for energy and growth. Genetic disorders that affect cellular metabolism may cause an excess or deficit in nutrients and cofactors necessary for physical and brain function. Phenylketonuria (PKU) and congenital hypothyroidism are examples of metabolic conditions that can lead to intellectual and developmental disabilities.

Degenerative disorders

Children with degenerative disorders may seem typical at birth and meet usual developmental milestones for a time, but then they experience disruptions in skills, abilities and functions. Pediatric neurodegenerative diseases include: subacute sclerosing panencephalitis, neuronal ceroid lipofuscinosis, tuberous sclerosis with degeneration, west disease, idiopathic degenerative encephalopathy associated with infantile spasms, Werdnig-Hoffmann disease, hereditary spastic paraplegia. In some cases, the degenerative disorder may not be detected until the child is an adolescent or adult and starts to show symptoms or lose abilities.

Can children with developmental disabilities be helped?

I believe so. And the sooner, the better.

Studies show that early life experience and especially sensory input from the mother leads to neuroplasticity of the neuroendocrine stress response and influences cognitive function. Enhanced sensory stimulation can help blunt the hypothalamic-pituitary-adrenal axis leading to resilience to stress and improved learning and memory.

So yes, early infant stimulation can help children with developmental delays from birth traumas, autism and prematurity.

My first child was born 10 weeks premature with intrauterine growth retardation, weighing only two and a half pounds - which was 60% of their expected weight. Premature infants tend to be developmentally delayed and take a while to catch up.

I was very much interested in what we could do to help them develop but received no guidance from their pediatrician. In my first trimester, I was accepted into the UCLA graduate program to become a nurse practitioner but had to delay entrance because I birthed a premature baby who needed my attention. Fortunately, at the time, there was a nurse practitioner working in the neonatal intensive care unit at our county hospital who was developing protocols for early infant stimulation to teach parents.

I instituted her early infant stimulation protocols with my firstborn. Premies are aged by their due date not their actual birth date, to determine their development. Typically, preterm infants, age-corrected for prematurity, score on average, 10 points lower on IQ tests than full-term infants tested at comparable ages.

With consistent early infant stimulation, my child was developmentally caught up by six months of actual age - babbling, crawling and using their hands. Due to micro-ophthalmia which limited their vision, they walked a bit late at fourteen months, but was speaking in full sentences by eighteen months and reading before their fourth birthday.

In California where I birthed my first child, it wasn't until 1986 that the Early Intervention Program for Infants and Toddlers with Disabilities was enacted.

Early infant intervention works. Parents must be educated on how to help their children and motivated to do the work. As parents, we must become our child's best advocate so that they can develop to their fullest potential.

Early intervention may include speech therapy, physical therapy, occupational therapy, nutritional therapy, educational services and psychological therapy for the child and family.

Like all children with developmental disabilities, Christina will need extra help through her preschool and elementary school years. By the time Christina becomes a teenager, she will need to be well established in the educational system to receive the support she needs to flourish intellectually, physically, emotionally and socially.

My assessment of Christina is hypothalamus dysfunction with developmental delay secondary to birth injury.

Since Christina is still very young and has missed vital infant stimulation, we will need to support optimal hypothalamus function throughout her childhood.

Here's what Christina's healing plan looks like:

1. Hypothalamus support - 3gms Genesis Gold® mixed in applesauce or juice. Dose to increase as Christina grows. Genesis Gold® has been used safely in children since 2003.

2. Nutrition - Continue organic diet with a variety of fruits and colorful vegetables, high fiber carbohydrates, protein including eggs and dairy, healthy fats like avocados, nuts, seeds, cooking with olive oil.

3. Activity - Abdominal exercises to close her diastasis - encourage play including climbing and especially hanging and lifting her legs up to strengthen abdominal muscles. Balance exercises like helping Christina navigate across obstacles, balance beams, etc.. I encourage family activity to encourage Christina to be active.

4. Sleep - Preschoolers need 11-13 hours of sleep, which includes a nap. Establish a regular bedtime routine - warm bath, reading a book or two, songs, prayers and saying goodnight. Only use a pink nightlight if needed - pink light helps the pineal gland make melatonin, otherwise Christina's room is to be as dark as possible. Young children naturally wake up with the sun if they get enough sleep.

5. Developmental - Children's work is play, so providing developmentally appropriate toys and activities with next level toys available to help challenge Christina will help her develop. I order speech evaluation and therapy to help Christina express herself verbally. I also order occupational evaluation and therapy to help Christina develop fine motor skills and refine her gross motor skills.

6. Mindset - For children, it's the parents' mindset that counts. I support continual development of their parenting skills, as well as relief from care especially for Christina's mother who is also homeschooling their son.

Results

After a few months, Christina's development started to progress. She began to speak and was able to communicate her needs verbally. Overtime, she was able to draw and use scissors. She learned to ride a tricycle and balance on one foot.

I worked with this child and her family for nearly two decades.

Prior to puberty, Christina's midline weight gain concerned her parents as she was active but craved carbohydrates. Her bloodwork revealed early signs of insulin resistance. Christina went through a normal puberty and started menstruating at the age of 13. We were able to get her insulin resistance and weight under better control with an exercise program designed for young children. She began horseback riding which helped strengthen her core. She learned to ride a bike and worked with a personal trainer throughout her teens.

Over the years, we needed to attend to Christina's gut and be sure she stayed in balance with a variety of beneficial bacteria. Studies show that the gut microbiome in children with autism and learning disabilities tends to be out of balance. Keeping Christina's gut microbiome healthy helped with her learning and development.

Christina was homeschooled with support from developmental specialists. She was able to take care of her personal hygiene, cook meals and help with household chores including caring for her horse and dog. After menarche, we utilized Ayurvedic herbs which worked well to get Christina's HGBA1C down. Her mother worked hard to be sure that Christina got an adequate amount of protein and fat, and ate low glycemic index carbohydrates to keep her blood sugar under control.

By mid-teens, Christina's weight was within 5% of ideal for her height. She has good aerobic endurance and strength. Her coordination is still a bit challenged, but she is able to keep up with the rest of the family pursuing outdoor activities including skiing, hiking and mountain biking. Christina is dependent on her family as her mental capacity limits her ability to financially support herself or live on her own.

Part Three

How to Heal Your Hypothalamus

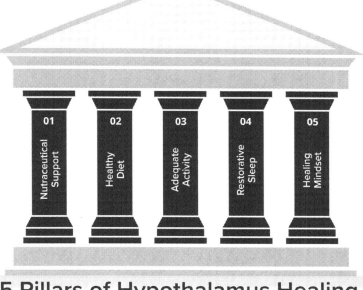

5 Pillars of Hypothalamus Healing

01	02	03	04	05
Nutraceutical Support	Healthy Diet	Adequate Activity	Restorative Sleep	Healing Mindset

Hypothalamus healing requires lifestyle changes - diet, exercise, sleep, attitude and nutraceutical support.

Chapter 10

Best Diet for your Hypothalamus

Unprotected by the blood brain barrier, your hypothalamus receives most of what it needs from your diet. Literally, you are what you eat.

If you eat a nutritious balanced diet, your hypothalamus can help you heal anything. If your diet is poor, your hypothalamus will not get what it needs and will become dysfunctional.

So, let's start with what you eat. Your hypothalamus is very sensitive to your nutritional intake - both macronutrients and micronutrients. Macronutrients are carbohydrates, fats and protein. Micronutrients are vitamins, minerals and co-factors, including amino acids and fatty acids.

Calories are units of energy from your food. You burn calories just by being alive and then more with activity. The more metabolically active your body is, the more calories you need.

Lean body mass is more metabolically active than body fat. Due to higher muscle mass, men tend to need more calories than women. Growing children need more calories per pound than adults. As we age, we become more metabolically sluggish and need less calories.

Your basal metabolic rate (BMR) is how much energy you expend. The most precise way to measure BMR is in a laboratory setting where you breathe into a mask called a calorimeter, which calculates your rate of breathing and uses it to measure how many calories you burn at rest.

To maintain your weight, your caloric intake must match your energy expenditure. To lose weight, you must consume less calories than you expend or expend more calories than you consume. Foods are not created equally - calorie wise. Carbohydrates provide pure caloric energy, while it's harder for your body to break down fat and protein into glucose for energy.

What's the best diet for hypothalamus health?

The best diet for hypothalamus health is the Mediterranean diet. In multiple studies, the Mediterranean diet has been shown to be the best anti-aging diet, hormone balancing diet and weight loss diet. Study after study rates the Mediterranean diet as the most effective in lowering the risk of cardiovascular disease, diabetes and cancer.

The worst diet for hypothalamus health is SAD - the Standard American Diet - which is too high in trans-fats, sugar, starches and too low in vegetables. Most of my patients come to me, having experimented with many different diets - vegan, vegetarian, paleo, keto and intermittent fasting - very few are still consuming a standard American diet.

It may seem that I'm biased in my preference for the Mediterranean diet being an Italian married to a Greek. Yes, I was raised on a Mediterranean diet. But in my teens, I began to eat ultra-low-fat fearing dietary fat would cause body fat. At the time, the American Medical Association supported a low fat diet as the best means to lower the risk of cardiovascular disease.

I was even a vegetarian for seven years - a healthy vegetarian who ate lots of vegetables, legumes, whole grains and avoided sugar and white flour like the plague. Yet, I still tried to follow a low fat diet. So you can imagine that I wasn't getting nearly enough essential fats or protein. Clearly, being a vegetarian was not the best diet for my hypothalamus as I was amenorrheic (no periods), had adult acne, dry brittle hair, plus I was hyperactive, insomniac, moody and constantly craved sugar with frequent bouts of hypoglycemia.

In my early thirties, I saw my internist who ran basic blood work and raved about my low cholesterol at 130. But I was alarmed. With my ultra-low HDL under 25, I was setting myself up for cardiovascular issues. And without periods, I was setting myself up for osteoporosis.

So, I went back to my roots and started eating a Mediterranean diet. I consumed at least 30% of my calories as fat - lots of olive oil, nuts, seeds, avocados and whole fat dairy. Immediately, my sugar cravings disappeared. Within a couple of months, my hair, skin and nails improved. While I didn't sleep through the night nor get my periods back until I started taking nutraceutical hypothalamus support, I felt better with more stable blood sugar and my cholesterol improved dramatically (total 190, HDL 90). I was very happy with those results.

At the base of the Mediterranean diet is plant foods - vegetables, fruits, legumes, whole grains. It also includes some dairy, mainly as cultured products like yogurt and cheeses. There's a lot of olive oil, plus nuts and seeds. It also contains animal protein coming from eggs, fish, poultry, and a little bit of red meat. At the very top of the Mediterranean diet pyramid is sugar - yes, it's okay to have a little bit if the rest of your diet is balanced. And of course, red wine. Red wine is rich in antioxidants, particularly cardio-protective resveratrol.

The Mediterranean diet offers such a wide variety of foods that you can actually find something you like to eat. No, it's not a lot of pasta and pizza but whole plant foods like vegetables. You really need to eat a variety of colorful produce. The color in the fruits and vegetables - purple, red, orange, yellow, green - is where the antioxidants exist.

So many of my health conscious patients eat too little variety. They may eat only five or six foods, which is not enough variety to get the micronutrients the hypothalamus needs and to prevent food sensitivities.

A bland diet is deficient in nutrients. So, limit white flour, white sugar, white potatoes and white rice. The more colorful your diet, the more antioxidants you get.

Carbohydrates = Energy

Carbohydrates are your energy food. If you choose your carbs wisely, you will get enough fiber to keep your gut healthy. Your intestinal microbiome depends on the fiber you consume for energy. Plus your microbiome uses fiber to produce protective short chain fatty acids.

Choose whole grains over processed grains. When grains are processed down to pale flour, fatty acid rich bran and gut healthy fiber are lost. All that's left is starch which converts to sugar very quickly. Starchy foods are high on the glycemic index.

The glycemic index (GI) of a food measures how fast it is turned to blood sugar compared to consuming pure glucose. Glucose has a GI of 100, fructose has a GI of 25 and sucrose— which is a blend of the previous two—has a GI of 65. Anything over 50 is considered high glycemic. All the white starchy carbs and sweets are high glycemic. Low glycemic index carbs include legumes, vegetables and most fruits.

The way you prepare your foods can help. Adding fat and protein to a starchy high glycemic carb, lowers its glycemic index. Pasta dressed with olive oil and Parmesan will slow down the absorption of the starch, which will lower its glycemic index. If you are obese, insulin resistant, diabetic, have high triglycerides or too many small particle LDL cholesterol, you would want to eat low glycemic index carbs and avoid high glycemic index carbs.

Paying attention to glycemic index is important but more important is how many carbohydrates you consume based on your activity level and body fat percentage. If you're a lean active athlete, you need more carbs. If you're obese and sedentary, you need much less.

Does that mean that you can't eat any sugars at all? Of course not. I eat sugar occasionally. Fruit is a great source of natural sugar and also contains fiber and antioxidants. Some fruits are lower glycemic than others. Berries are low glycemic index. Bananas are moderate glycemic index. While I'm not a fan of bananas, I do love watermelon, which is a high glycemic index fruit. If you eat high glycemic fruit, it's best to balance it with protein and fat to lower the glycemic index.

For instance, I like eating prosciutto with Tuscan melon. That's very Italian. What I keep on hand all the time are protein and fat rich nuts and seeds to keep my blood sugar stable so that I don't get a rise from the fruit then bottom out and have a hypoglycemic reaction. Since I began supporting my hypothalamus nutraceutically, I rarely have hypoglycemic reactions.

What about alcohol?

Red wine is included in the Mediterranean diet. Studies show that moderate alcohol consumption can reduce your risk of diabetes, ischemic stroke and heart disease. What's moderate? One serving of alcohol daily for women and two servings for men. A serving is one 4 oz glass of wine or 12 oz of beer or 1 oz of hard liquor.

Yet, it matters if you drink (or eat) emotionally. When you use a substance to change the way you feel, like calming down your anxiety, you're trying to treat neurotransmitter imbalances. If you have a genetic tendency for addiction, you may develop a substance abuse disorder. Being conscious of why you're drinking alcohol may help you be more moderate.

What about caffeine?

Your consumption of caffeine should be less than 400mg per day. An eight ounce cup of coffee has 95mg of caffeine.

Caffeine can be found in coffee, tea and chocolate. Studies show that coffee has unique benefits. Coffee may lower the risk of type 2 diabetes, support brain health, lower the risk of depression, protect against liver conditions, support heart health and possibly increase longevity. Tea is also a great anti-inflammatory beverage. The problem for most coffee and tea drinkers is using sweeteners including dairy alternative creamers. And the amount of caffeine they need to consume to function.

I've always had a lot of energy in the morning. What coffee helps me do is to actually slow down and relax. My grandmother, who influenced my childhood and my husband's grandmother, who I spent time with at the end of her life, sat down to drink their coffee. Coffee was me-time for them. Coffee is me-time for me. I drink my coffee in an actual cup, sit down and relax with it.

Remember, consume everything in moderation.

Everybody's different on how they deal with the foods they eat. If you find that you crave a lot of sugar or other unhealthy foods, ask yourself: Is it an emotional or physical craving? Because if you need the energy, eating a yam is just as effective as a candy bar.

Now, I do eat chocolate - antioxidant rich dark chocolate. Chocolate's great at boosting serotonin. I used to use chocolate for my PMS. A couple days before my period, when I felt irritable, I'd have some dark chocolate but I'd sit down with it and treat it like medicine, just an ounce to try to get my serotonin up. And it usually worked.

Food can be your medicine, it can also be your pleasure, but if you're using it emotionally, it may lead to an eating disorder and you may have some weight issues. So, think about the reason you eat, not just about what you eat.

Is emotional eating always emotional?

Studies show that emotional eating is very common. An analysis of over 5000 adults found that over 20% eat emotionally, with the prevalence higher in young white women.

Physiologically, hunger is hormonally regulated. There are two main hunger pathways: the homeostatic pathway and the hedonic pathway. The homeostatic pathway controlled by our hypothalamus is your biological hunger pathway and is driven by the need for energy in calories. The hedonic eating is pleasure-driven and uses emotional stimuli to "bypass" the physical hunger/satisfaction signals.

Factors that disrupt the hypothalamic appetite regulation include sleep disturbances, high stress levels; and medical conditions like obesity, diabetes, PCOS. Insulin resistance and inflammation at the hypothalamic level are the common links affecting appetite and satiety.

Mental health conditions that disrupt levels of neurotransmitters can also cause appetite changes.

Physiologically disrupted appetite can trigger emotional eating. Having strong emotional connections to food and behavior patterns can trigger emotional eating.

Places and psychological conditions can also trigger emotional eating. Holidays, vacations, proximity to certain restaurants, exposure to food marketing, and major life shifts can lead to increased emotional eating. Emotional eating can also be a symptom of mood disorders like anxiety and depression. Many emotional eaters have experienced significant adverse childhood events.

If you are an emotional eater, you may need professional help to change your emotional eating to physiological eating based on energy and micro-nutrient needs

What if you need to lose weight?

Well, if you need to lose some body fat, I've found that an insulin resistant diet can be very effective. For my insulin resistant, diabetic and obese patients, I developed a specific insulin resistant diet.

I have them limit their sugars and starches intake. In fact, they don't even get grains and starchy vegetables in the first phase of my insulin resistant diet. By restricting carbohydrates, we are attempting to get their bodies to burn their fat stores for energy and start the process of weight loss.

In phase two, they can add some carbs like brown rice or quinoa. If their weight doesn't change and they're not bloated or craving more sugar after adding carbs, their body has increased insulin sensitivity.

Sometimes when you eat starches, you just want more. If they're at that point where they keep desiring more, they can add one serving a day and then stay there for a while. If they continue to lose weight, great, then they try two servings a day. This simply means that they've raised their metabolism through the insulin resistant diet and, of course, with nutraceutical hypothalamus support.

Their metabolism is higher now, so they go into their fat stores for energy because they're not getting all they need from their diet. As soon as they lose all the body fat that they need to lose, then we can start adding even more carbohydrates according to how much energy they're expending.

If you're really sedentary, you're probably not expending that much energy. It's important that you're eating for your body, so it can get all the nutrients it needs and enough energy but not so much that you store excess body fat.

When should you eat?

Everybody is different. Some people can go a long time without eating. I believe you need to break your fast and eat breakfast. Studies have shown that your metabolism is higher when you break your fast early in the morning. Breakfast is important to jumpstart daily energy expenditure. A randomized clinical trial showed that skipping breakfast adversely affects circadian gene expression (messes up your day/night cycle) and correlates with increased postprandial glycemic response (higher blood sugar after you eat).

Now breakfast is not just coffee and toast or a piece of fruit. Like all your meals, breakfast should include low glycemic carbohydrates, fat and protein. My go-to breakfast is whole milk yogurt or cottage cheese with berries and homemade granola or high fiber cereal. The cultured dairy is rich in protein, has some fat, plus the granola has fat from coconut oil, nuts and seeds and carbohydrates from the whole grain and berries. It's a complete little meal.

Since it was hard for my patients to figure out exactly what they needed to eat and because I believe that most people do not get enough protein to maintain lean body mass to be metabolically active nor the right kind

of fat for healthy cells and hormone production, I created my DMAR®
Nutritional Plan for Wellness. It's yours in the resources section along with
my Insulin Resistant Diet.

DMAR® NUTRITIONAL WELLNESS

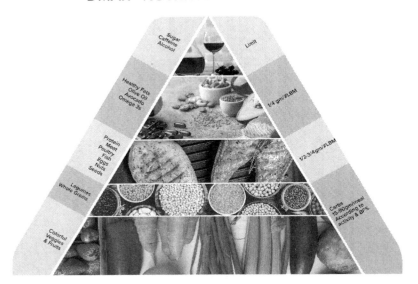

D. MARAGOPOULOS © 2023

What's the best time to eat?

Eating a large breakfast, a substantial lunch and a very light dinner early in
the evening aligns with our innate 24-hour clock or circadian rhythm when
our bodies are most efficient at metabolizing meals in the morning and early
afternoon.

Studies show that people who eat most of their calories early in the day, lose
more weight and have greater improvements in their blood sugar, cholesterol
levels and other metabolic risk factors compared to people who eat most of
their calories later in the day. They also burn more fat and experience less
hunger when following an early-eating schedule.

Should you eat two, three or five times a day? Again, it depends on what your body needs. People with super high energy may need to eat more frequently while others may need to eat less frequently, but people who only eat once or even twice a day tend to have a slower metabolism.

I've consulted with a lot of overweight people who don't eat all day long yet eat all evening. Eating late at night is the worst time to consume large amounts of calories because you're not going to utilize those calories for energy since you'll soon be going to bed.

You can only store 400 calories worth of sugar in the form of glycogen in your liver and muscles. The calories you consume that you do not use as energy are stored in your fat cells. So, if you eat your 2000 calories after dusk and can only store 400 for energy, the rest goes into your fat cells and you don't release it from your fat cells very easily.

It's better to spread those calories out during the day. If you really want to lose weight, avoid eating the majority of your calories at night. In fact, you should eat less than a third of your calories after dusk, even less would be better. Your mid-day meal should be your biggest meal. Your breakfast should be your second largest and dinner, the smallest.

What about people who snack between meals? If you have a very high metabolism or you're a very young child, you probably do need to eat more frequently. But if you have SIBO; small intestinal bacterial overgrowth and you're eating more than every four hours, you're keeping the ileocecal valve open, which allows more bacteria to migrate from your colon into your small intestine. You need to let your gastrointestinal tract digest and absorb for at least four hours before you eat again.

What about intermittent fasting?

I recommend circadian fasting. Don't eat after dark. Break your fast in the morning and consume your food during the daylight. Circadian fasting works best to keep your hormones and metabolism functioning in natural healthy rhythms.

Traditional intermittent fasting, where you don't break your fast until later in the afternoon and eat only in a 6-8 hour window, may work to lose weight in the beginning but you will certainly gain it back. Messing with your natural circadian rhythms disrupts hypothalamus function. Your hypothalamus goes into survival mode and tells your body to store fat.

Following the natural circadian rhythm promotes a healthy metabolism. You weren't meant to be eating in the middle of the night. Does that mean to never eat after dark? Of course not. Just don't eat the majority of your calories after dark.

When you eat counts as much as what you eat.

Protein = New You

Protein provides amino acids which are your body's building blocks. Out of twenty amino acids, nine are essential, meaning you must get them from your diet as your body does not make them. Some amino acids are considered conditionally essential because the body cannot synthesize them in sufficient quantities during certain physiological periods of growth, including pregnancy, adolescence, or recovery from trauma.

During states of inadequate intake of essential amino acids such as vomiting or low appetite, symptoms may appear, including depression, anxiety, insomnia, fatigue, weakness and even stunting the growth of young children. These symptoms are mostly caused by a lack of protein synthesis in the body because of the lack of essential amino acids. Sufficient quantities of amino acids are necessary to produce neurotransmitters, hormones, grow muscle, bone and other tissues.

Complete protein sources include all the essential amino acids. Animal proteins are complete - meat, seafood, poultry, eggs and dairy products. While soy and peas are complete plant-based protein sources, you have to eat a lot to get enough essential amino acids.

Other plant-based sources of protein such as beans, nuts and certain grains are considered incomplete proteins because they lack one or more of the essential amino acids. If you're a vegetarian, consuming a variety of protein rich plant foods can help ensure you're getting all nine essential amino acids.

*Essential Amino Acids

Essential means that our bodies cannot produce these amino acids, so we must get them from our diet. Essential amino acids include histidine, isoleucine, leucine, lysine, methionine, phenylalanine, threonine, tryptophan and valine.

Nonessential Amino Acids

Nonessential means that our bodies can produce the amino acid, even if we do not get it from the food we eat. Nonessential amino acids include alanine, arginine, asparagine, aspartic acid, cysteine, glutamic acid, glutamine, glycine, proline, serine and tyrosine.

Conditional Amino Acids

Conditional amino acids are usually not essential, except in times of illness and stress. Conditional amino acids include arginine, cysteine, glutamine, tyrosine, glycine, ornithine, proline and serine.

Make sure you're getting an adequate amount of protein. What is an adequate amount? You need at least one half gram of protein per pound of lean body mass.

Amino Acids

Name of Amino Acid	Single Letter Denotation	Function
Alanine	(A)	Used to break down tryptophan and vitamin B-6, is a source of energy for muscles and the central nervous system, the immune system and helps the body use sugars.
Arginine	(R)	Assists in wound healing , helps remove excess ammonia from the body, stimulates immune function , and promotes secretion of several hormones, including glucagon, insulin , and growth hormone.
Asparagine	(N)	Helps to break down toxic ammonia within cells, is important for protein modification, and is needed for neurotransmitter synthesis.
Aspartic Acid	(D)	Used to break down tryptophan and vitamin B-6, is a source of energy for muscles and the central nervous system, the immune system and helps the body use sugars.
Cysteine	(C)	Important for making protein like collagen and beta-keratin - the main protein in nails, skin, and hair.
Glutamine	(Q)	The most abundant and versatile amino acid that's important for removing excess ammonia from your cells, helps your immune system and brain function and aids in intestinal nutrient absorption .
Glutamic Acid	(E)	Used to form proteins and turns into glutamate which helps nerve cells in the brain send and receive information.
Glycine	(G)	Is a precursor for a variety of important metabolites such as glutathione, porphyrins, purines, and creatine. Glycine acts as neurotransmitter in central nervous system and in the peripheral tissues has antioxidant, anti-inflammatory, cryoprotective, and immunomodulatory.
Histidine	(H)	Essential amino acid used to produce histamine, a neurotransmitter that is vital to immune response, digestion, sexual function, and sleep-wake cycles. Histidine is critical for maintaining the myelin sheath, a protective barrier that surrounds your nerve cells.
Isoleucine	(I)	Essential branched-chain amino acid (BCAA) is involved in muscle metabolism and is important for immune function, hemoglobin production, and energy regulation
Leucine	(L)	Essential branched-chain amino acid (BCAA) critical for protein synthesis and muscle repair and helps regulate blood sugar levels, stimulate wound healing, and produce growth hormones.
Lysine	(K)	Essential amino acid plays major roles in protein synthesis, calcium absorption, and the production of hormones and enzymes, as well as energy production, immune function, and the production of collagen and elastin.
Methionine	(M)	Essential amino acid plays an important role in metabolism and detoxification and is necessary for tissue growth and the absorption of zinc and selenium.
Phenylalanine	(F)	Essential amino acid used for neurotransmitter production - tyrosine, dopamine, epinephrine, norepinephrine
Proline	(P)	Plays important roles in protein synthesis and structure, metabolism, nutrition, wound healing, antioxidative reactions, and immune responses.
Serine	(S)	Plays a role in the biosynthesis of proteins, phospholipids, purines, pyrimidines, the amino acids cysteine and glycine.
Threonine	(T)	Essential amino acid that is part of structural proteins like collagen and elastin and plays a role in fat metabolism and immune function.
Tryptophan	(W)	Essential amino acid that is precursor to serotonin which regulates your mood, appetite, and sleep.
Tyrosine	(Y)	Essential component for the production of neurotransmitters - epinephrine, norepinephrine, and dopamine as well as helps produce melanin, the pigment responsible for hair and skin color.
Valine	(V)	Essential branched-chain amino acids (BCAA) helps stimulate muscle growth and regeneration and is involved in energy production.

How do you know what your lean body mass is?

To calculate your lean body mass (LBM), you need to calculate your body fat percentage and multiple it by your weight. That gives you your pounds of body fat. Subtract your pounds of body fat from your weight to get your LBM.

The most accurate way to measure your body fat is with underwater weighing, but it's difficult and not commonly done. You can also use calipers on different areas of your body to measure body fat. I've had my body fat measured in all these ways and the online calculators are pretty accurate unless you're an athlete with very low body fat.

You can use an online calculator which asks for your height, weight and some measurements like neck, waist and hips to determine your body fat percentage and pounds of LBM.

My lean body mass is about a hundred pounds, so I need to eat at least 50 grams of protein a day to maintain it. If I eat less than that, I'm literally going to consume my own muscles to make hormones, repair tissues and produce enzymes. Especially as a menopausal woman, I do not want to lose muscle tissue and become metabolically inactive.

How do you know you're eating enough protein?

For animal protein, the size of a deck of cards, or about what fits in the palm of your hand is three to four ounces and is usually anywhere from 20 to 25 grams of protein. An egg has nine grams of protein. Legumes have any-where from five to 14 grams of protein per serving, which is usually a cup, but there's carbs in legumes that you need to take into account.

Once you know your lean body mass, you can calculate how much body fat you need to lose and lean body mass you might need to gain to determine how much protein you need to eat.

Before the scale moves too much, you will notice you're getting thinner. If you're active and eating better, you'll be losing body fat. Also, you may gain lean body mass, which weighs two and a half times more than fat. So, your scale may not change much but your measurements smaller.

That's more important. If you look the way you'd like to look and you feel good, it doesn't really matter what the scale says.

If you're an athlete, you need at least three quarters of a gram of protein per pound of LBM. When I was a competitive triathlete, I actually weighed more than I do now because I had more lean body mass, but I was smaller because lean body mass is heavier than body fat.

Fat = Healthy Cells

You need fat in your diet for healthy cell membranes, neurons, hormones, immune and brain function. Yet, dietary fat is not created equally. While fats are made up of carbon, hydrogen and oxygen molecules, the types of bonds between the molecules determines if the fat is saturated, unsaturated or a trans-fat.

Most foods contain a mix of fats. Animal products have more saturated fats while plants and fish have more unsaturated fats. Saturated fats like butter are solid at room temperature. Unsaturated fats like olive oil are liquid at room temperature.

Saturated fatty acids are used by cells as building blocks for membrane lipids, stored in lipid droplets or used to modify proteins. But consuming too much saturated fats can stiffen the normally flexible membrane of the endoplasmic reticulum and impair its function. Remember the endoplasmic reticulum is a cellular organelle that processes protein to create vital biochemicals and structures.

Man-made trans-fats are the most dangerous and should be avoided. Trans-fats are created by adding hydrogen to vegetable oils called a partially hydrogenated oil, which is highly inflammatory.

The majority of your dietary fat should be unsaturated but you must pay attention to how you cook with it, even the safer polyunsaturated fats. Heating oil to the smoking point may decrease the amount of polyunsaturated fatty acids because of oxidative degradation.

There are two types of unsaturated fats: monounsaturated fatty acids (MUFAs) and polyunsaturated fatty acids (PUFAs). Monounsaturated fatty acids are found in plant and nut oils, as well as animal fats. Omega-9s are MUFA's. Polyunsaturated fatty acids are found in plant oils and nuts and seeds, as well as fatty fish. Omega-3s and Omega-6s are PUFAs.

"Omega" refers to the tail end of the fat molecule. The numbers "3-6-9" refer to how many carbon atoms from the end the double bond is.

Since the human body can't produce Omega-3s, these fats are referred to as "essential fats," which means that you have to get them from your diet.

Omega-3 fatty acids make up part of cell membranes, ease inflammation, help protect the heart from potentially deadly erratic rhythms, inhibit the formation of dangerous clots in the bloodstream and lower levels of triglycerides.

There are many types of Omega-3 fats that differ based on their chemical shape and size. Here are the three most common:

- Eicosapentaenoic acid (EPA): This 20-carbon fatty acid's main function is to produce chemicals called eicosanoids, which help reduce inflammation. EPA improves estrogen metabolism and may help reduce symptoms of depression.

- Docosahexaenoic acid (DHA): A 22-carbon fatty acid, DHA makes up about 8% of brain weight and contributes to brain development and function. DHA is vital in fetal and infant brain development.

- Alpha-linolenic acid (ALA): This 18-carbon fatty acid can be converted into EPA and DHA, although the process is not very efficient. ALA appears to benefit the heart, immune system and nervous system.

Omega-6 fatty acids lower harmful LDL cholesterol, boost protective HDL and help keep blood sugar in check by improving the body's sensitivity to insulin.

Omega-6s have gotten a bad rap because the body can convert the most common Omega-6, linolenic acid, into another fatty acid called arachidonic acid. Arachidonic acid is a building block for molecules that promote inflammation, blood clotting and the constriction of blood vessels. When your body is injured, it needs a pro-inflammatory response.

Unfortunately, the inflammatory Western diet has too much Omega-6s and not nearly enough Omega-3s. Humans evolved on a diet with a ratio of 1:1 Omega-6 to Omega-3 essential fatty acids. In modern Western diets, the ratio is often greater than 15:1.

Omega-9 fatty acids represent one of the main mono-unsaturated fatty acids (MUFAs), which is found in plant and animal sources. Our bodies can make Omega-9s but not enough for optimal health, so Omega 9s are partially essential fatty acids. MUFAs have several health benefits, including anti-inflammatory and anti-cancer characteristics.

PUFAs help stimulate skin and hair growth, maintain bone health, regulate metabolism and maintain the reproductive system.

The ideal Omega-3:Omega-6:Omega-9 dietary ratio is 2:1:1.

Omega-3 sources: Oily fish such as salmon, herring, mackerel and sardines, fish and flaxseed oil, flaxseeds, walnuts and chia seeds.

Omega-6 sources: Safflower oil, sunflower oil, corn oil, soybean oil, sunflower seeds, walnuts and pumpkin seeds.

Omega-9 sources: Olive oil, cashew nut oil, almond oil, avocado oil, peanut oil, almonds, cashews and walnuts.

How much fat do you need?

At least half as much fat as protein or one quarter gram of fat per pound of lean body mass. Fat is higher in calories at 9 calories per gram versus 4 calories per gram of protein or carbohydrates. So, fat won't take as much space on your plate.

You need both saturated and unsaturated fats in your diet. Up to one third of your fat intake can be saturated and the rest unsaturated.

The majority of my plate has plant foods - half is vegetables, one third is fruits, legumes or whole grains while the rest is protein with a little bit of fat. Normally, I don't put the fat on the side, instead I drizzle olive oil over everything. If I'm eating chicken or salmon, I eat the skin. Nuts and seeds on my salad count as some of the fat too.

It takes time and reading of labels to understand the nutritional value of foods. Knowing how much protein, fat and carbohydrates your food choices contain is important. You'll start to get a gist of it eventually. Just make sure that you're getting enough fat for healthy cells and hormones, protein for healthy tissues and muscles and lots of colorful carbohydrates for energy and antioxidants.

The more you understand about your food, the better choices you can make to help your hypothalamus function optimally.

My DMAR® Path to Nutritional Wellness provides the formulas you need to figure out the macronutrient requirements for your body.

Chapter 11

Activity for Hypothalamus Health

My grandmother rarely sat down. From dawn until bedtime, Nana was busy hustling about the house, cleaning, doing laundry, going up and down the stairs and cooking three meals a day for us. In the afternoon, she watched her soap operas while standing to fold and iron. Nana would only sit down and relax at meals or whenever she had a cup of coffee and she maintained her slim figure well after menopause.

Did you know that being sedentary is like smoking today? Yes, a sedentary lifestyle increases your risk of life threatening diseases, just like smoking does.

If you don't move your body, you age prematurely, which predisposes you to chronic illnesses, including cardiovascular disease, diabetes, metabolic syndrome and cancer. Being active helps to keep your hormones balanced. When you're active, you're telling your hypothalamus that life is good, so there's no need to lower your metabolism and store unnecessary body fat. So it is vital that you get moving.

Before technology and machines, we had to be active to survive. We planted and tended our own crops. We cut our own firewood, tended livestock, and baked our own bread. We washed our laundry by hand, drew our water from streams and wells and carried loads of weight throughout the day - all of which strengthened our bodies.

For years, I had horses. Being an equestrian is a physical activity even if you're not riding. I mucked stalls, transported about 50 pounds of manure every day from the corral to the manure pile, picked up heavy bags of grain and threw heavy flakes of hay into feeders. It's physical work to take care of livestock. Within six months after my last horse passed away, I noticed that I wasn't as strong and toned, so I had to do weight resistance exercises for the first time in my life.

If you want to be healthy, maintain your muscle tone, strength, flexibility and endurance, you need to be active. You can swim, row, or ride a bicycle. You can walk, hike, or run. You can also dance to get your body moving.

Activity is important to hypothalamus health. Being sedentary is not a natural human state. You need to move your body. In our developed society, we don't use our bodies like we did before technology. We're not as physically active, so we have to do some kind of exercise.

Studies show that exercising can increase your longevity and the quality of your life by slowing down diseases of old age. Exercise increases muscle mass, which is important for your metabolic health as muscles are the most metabolically active tissues in your body.

I like to think of exercise as a three legged stool; aerobic, strength and flexibility.

Aerobic Exercise

Anything you like to do that increases your heart rate is aerobic exercise. How do you know your heart rate is up? Besides wearing a heart monitor, try

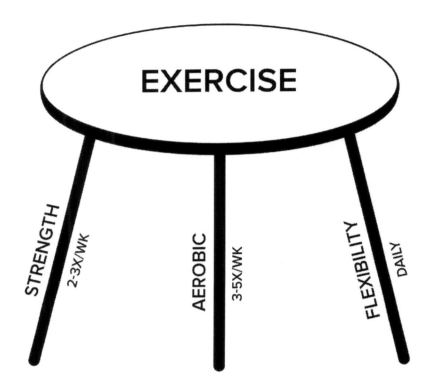

STRENGTH 2-3X/WK

AEROBIC 3-5X/WK

FLEXIBILITY DAILY

D. MARAGOPOULOS © 2023

singing while you're exercising and then increase your speed. When you get to the point where you can't sing because you're breathing harder, you're in the aerobic zone. Just keep going.

One of the best exercises to get the beneficial effects of aerobics is high intensity training (HIT). A cardiovascular surgeon measured the effect of HIT on the cardiopulmonary function of athletes compared to non-athletes.

The athletes needed way more time in the aerobic zone to improve their cardiopulmonary function because they already had great cardiopulmonary function. But the rest of the subjects didn't need that much time. In fact, all they needed was three minutes a week. Only three 20 second bursts of speed three times a week improved their cardiopulmonary function, increased insulin sensitivity, lowered cholesterol after 12 weeks. And they lost body fat.

To test this minimal HIT theory, I participated in a little experiment with about a dozen of my patients from 35 to 70 years of age. All of them wanted to lose some weight and some had insulin resistance. After eight weeks, they all had positive changes in their blood work and experienced weight loss, particularly fat loss as they noted their waist measurements going down. The ones who combined my insulin resistant diet with HIT had the most benefits.

So what does HIT look like? For me, since I've put so many miles on my body being a triathlete, I don't run anymore. I do power walking, hiking and cycling. Power walking up a hill is the best way for me to get in the aerobic zone. And it's pretty easy to do. I do a ten-minute warm-up. It takes me a little bit longer to warm up because as a retired athlete, I have increased cardiopulmonary capacity. When I get to a hill, I walk as fast as I can for twenty seconds. I know I've reached my aerobic zone when I can't sing while power walking. Once I reach the top of the hill, I walk slowly back down for about one minute. Then I do the sprint again two more times. I do HIT three times a week, skipping a day between.

My HIT formula is quite easy to do. It does not have to be walking or running. It could be rowing. You could do HIT on the elliptical. You could do HIT in swim bursts, while cycling or during dance aerobics. The goal is to move as fast as you can. You could jump rope for your HIT activity. Whatever it takes to get your heart rate up for 20 seconds, three repetitions, three times a week. Just make sure you slow your pace in between for one to two minutes. Then cool down for at least five to 10 minutes afterwards.

While aerobic exercise is one leg of the exercise stool, if you want to increase your endurance, you need to do one long slow distance (LSD) a week. For my LSD, I like to mountain bike or hike for at least an hour or two. You don't go into the fat burning zone until after 45 minutes of exercise. Remember, for endurance and to burn fat, your LSD doesn't have to be so vigorous that you can't keep up a conversation or sing.

Strength Training

The second leg of the exercise stool is strength training. You've got to use your muscles. Does that mean you have to lift heavy weights? Not necessarily. You can do calisthenics, using your own body weight as resistance. I like to do triceps dips off a chair where you scoot your bottom off the seat, keep your legs straight, hands on the seat and bend your elbows, dipping your bottom down and then push yourself up. It's a great way to tone the triceps.

Plank pose is another great weight resistance exercise which tones arms, back and abdomen. You can use bands for resistance and of course, actual weights like dumbbells or weight resistance machines. Just be sure you use proper technique so you don't strain your joints. Do some type of weight resistance exercise at least a couple times a week.

Weight resistance helps to build muscle and bone, and it can also raise your metabolism. Building muscle strength can help with balance and prevent falls.

Flexibility

The third leg of the exercise stool is maintaining your flexibility. That means stretching. You should be doing general stretches on your whole body and pay attention to any parts of your body that are particularly tight. If you have a stiff back, neck and tight hamstrings, work on those parts and keep stretching. As you get older, you lose flexibility first. So you must keep limber.

Be sure you hold stretches for at least fifteen seconds. Static stretching in which you hold the stretch can be combined with pulse stretching in which you gently stretch and release trying to go deeper and deeper. But be careful. If you're experiencing any pain especially in a joint, don't push the stretch. Listen to your body. Yoga is a great way to learn how to stretch.

Flexibility, strength training and aerobic exercise are the three keys to exercise.

Let's say you have a sedentary lifestyle where you have to sit in front of a computer eight hours a day, five days a week. You need to get out of that chair at least once every half hour for at least five minutes, and move. Do some brisk walks and stretching. Just get up and move around. If you can stand up, that's better. Standing work desks may help. Most of the time, I work on my tablet on a countertop so that I can stand instead of sitting. But I still take breaks every half hour to get my blood flowing and to stretch.

Studies have shown that doing thirty minutes of walking daily can help you lose weight. But you don't have to do it all at once. Three ten-minute walking sessions a day works. Just get those steps in. Most people burn 30-40 calories per 1,000 steps they walk, meaning they'll burn 300 to 400 calories by walking 10,000 steps. The specific number of calories burned in one hour of walking depends on your body weight. The more you weigh, the more calories you burn per step.

Your hypothalamus talks to your muscles. Inter-communication between the hypothalamus and skeletal muscle plays a key role in the preservation of physiological functions - locomotor activity, appetite, cognition and health.

The more you move, the better. The more active you are, the happier your hypothalamus will be.

Chapter 12

Your Hypothalamus Needs Sleep

S leep disorders plague our modern society. Over the last century, more and more of the earth is lit up at night. Since digital technology has found its way into every home and nearly every hand, we are exposed to blue screen lights long after dark. And stress can seriously disrupt your sleep.

I never got much sleep in my youth. From the age of 18 to 38, I maybe got 3-5 hours a night. Plus I had somnambulance - sleep walking. It was not unusual for me to wake up in the middle of the street with my Great Dane at my side watching over me. It wasn't until I started supporting my hypothalamus nutraceutically that I finally began sleeping through the night.

Sleep is vital for your health. Getting enough sleep helps to ensure that your immune system is functioning normally. Sleep helps your brain function well and your hormones stay balanced. Your hypothalamus controls your circadian rhythm and it's adversely affected by lack of sleep.

Let's say you work graveyard shifts or you don't go to bed on time. Perhaps you're studying too late, watching television on your devices, not shutting off the lights, or just not getting enough sleep in the dark to make adequate melatonin. Studies show that missing sleep can adversely affect your cell's sensitivity to insulin and may lead to prediabetes.

When you've been sleep deprived for long enough, you can develop hypothalamic dysfunction. And yes, hypothalamus dysfunction also causes sleep disorders.

The amount of sleep you need is determined by your age. The younger you are, the more sleep you need. The older you are, the less sleep you need. But the minimum for most people is at least seven to nine hours of sleep per night for healthy hypothalamus function.

Sleep requirements for healthy hypothalamus function:

13-18 y/o need at least 8-10 hrs of sleep

18-60 y/o need at least 7 hrs of sleep

>60 y/o need at least 7-9 hrs of sleep

The key to your best sleep is darkness. The pink light at dusk blocks the blue light of day and tells your hypothalamus that night is coming. Your hypothalamus then induces your pineal gland to start producing melatonin.

If you don't produce enough melatonin at night, you're not going to sleep deeply. You may not fall asleep nor stay asleep. After dusk, you need to get off of your devices or wear blue blocking glasses when using them. It's best not to have the device in bed with you or the television on because the blue light from screens interfere with melatonin production and the depth of your sleep.

You want your room as dark as possible. Use light blocking shades or drapes on your windows to block street lights. Cover your digital clocks as well. You don't want any light at all in the room. If you need a light to get to the bathroom, something that's in the pink or red zone is okay, because it mimics dusk and prevents melatonin from bottoming out. White, blue or green lights are not good for deep sleep. If your child needs a nightlight, get a pink bulb and you both will sleep better.

Be sure your bed is super comfortable with comfy linens. Pay attention to your pajamas - not too heavy or too light for you. Being too cold or too hot will prevent deep sleep.

Make sure the room temperature is 60 to 70 degrees Fahrenheit, any warmer makes it difficult to make enough melatonin. Your hypothalamus needs it to be cooler for your pineal gland to produce enough melatonin and keep you asleep.

You may need ambient noise. Some people are disturbed by the noise around them or they can't sleep in the complete quiet. A white noise machine can be a really great investment to help to stay asleep. White noise can be ocean sounds or rain, whatever works for you to sleep.

Waking up with the rising sun can help your body get into a healthy circadian rhythm. Putting up night shades on your windows to completely darken your room will not allow natural light in the morning. You might want to get an alarm clock that uses natural light that turns on about the time that you need to wake up. A light alarm begins at least 15 to 30 minutes before you need to wake up and it gets brighter and brighter to wake you up.

You want to get sun exposure every day, at least 20 minutes of daylight to make enough serotonin to flux into melatonin at night and then to flux back into serotonin when it's daylight again. Light exposure is very important to maintaining proper circadian rhythms and for your mental health.

Your hypothalamus needs you to get enough sleep in the dark but you may have to use sleep aids to fall asleep. Hypothalamus nutraceutical support will help you fall asleep. It takes at least 90 days to reset your hypothalamus, so in the beginning, you may need help to relax your nervous system using GABA, valerian root, theanine or passion flower.

If you have to use sleep aids for long periods of time, then your body gets dependent on them. I usually recommend that my patients use my sleep cocktail for about three weeks to help reset their circadian rhythm until their hypothalamus can begin to heal. My favorite sleep cocktail includes slow release melatonin, homeopathic valerian root and passion flower. Once my patient's circadian rhythm is reset, they usually do pretty well. If they travel, get sick or have a sick child interfering with their sleep, they may need to revisit the sleep cocktail in order to help them fall back to sleep again.

We always discuss sleep training as well. Yes, adults may need sleep training too. That means you need a regular bedtime. It's okay to have an occasional late night, but as you get older, you're going to find that you suffer the next day if you stay up too late. That's because you're low on growth hormone which is produced at night. When you're younger, you can have late nights all weekend long and still be able to go to college classes on Monday without any problem. But it's harder to recover when you're older. If you're missing sleep during the week, you may have to have a longer sleep time on weekends in order to catch up. However, it's better to get the sleep your body needs on a regular basis.

If you stay up late all the time and not get enough sleep, your hypothalamus can't do its job properly. For your body, nocturnal mode is about getting your immune system to protect you. All your other hormones that are in high metabolic mode during the day are turned down at night.

In the working world, most janitors come in after office hours. Your hypothalamus needs you to turn everything else off in order to detox your body. That's why it's very common to experience difficulties sleeping when you eat a heavy meal before you go to bed. You may even wake up in the middle of the night because digestion interferes with sleep.

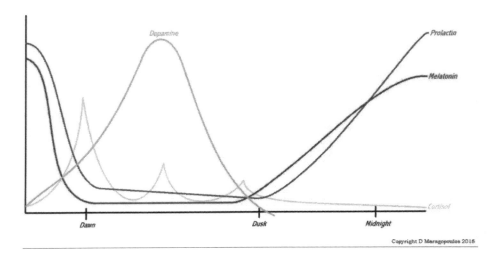

Sleep Training

In order to help my patients with insomnia, I've developed a step-by-step adult sleep training guide that I'm going to share with you. If you want to set a new sleep habit, you're going to have to do this for at least fourteen nights.

- **Develop a relaxing bedtime routine.** Start at dusk – that's when any digital blue light exposure will delay your melatonin production. No computer work or TV after dusk, for at least for fourteen nights straight. After that, you can use blue-light-blocking glasses if you must have screen time.

- **Tell your brain – specifically your hypothalamus – that it's time to go to sleep.** A hot bath before bed can help you relax. Add Epsom salts for even more muscle relaxation. Some calming essential oils like lavender can help trigger your brain chemistry to wind down. Get in your comfy pajamas, then curl up in bed and read a book or magazine. Don't read the news or scroll through social media. You need something relaxing.

  Perhaps you can add journaling to your nighttime routine. I like to record my reflections from the day; write down any insights and count my blessings on paper. When I say "journal," I'm not talking about writing down to-do lists. Don't get your brain revved up in bed. If you must create a to-do list for the next day, do it right after dinner and before you start your bedtime ritual. Don't bring your worries into bed.

- **Turn off all the lights.** Your bedroom must be completely dark - no lights in your bedroom whatsoever. No digital lights, no night lights, no television. If you have any lights on at night, you're effectively telling your hypothalamus that it's daytime. So your hypothalamus does not trigger your pineal gland to make adequate melatonin to keep you asleep.

- **Be sure your room temperature is just right.** Your hypothalamus needs to be signaled that it's nighttime by an adjustment of temperature too. Your bedroom temperature should be between 60-67 degrees Fahrenheit. Any cooler and you'll be cold and have trouble sleeping. Any warmer and you won't be able to sleep deeply. A cool bedroom temperature is especially important for pregnant women and nursing moms, perimenopausal and menopausal women and men going through andropause (the male equivalent of the change of life). If you're consistently cold at night, consider getting your thyroid function checked.

- **Use ambient noise to lull yourself into a deep sleep.** A white noise machine will do. What makes you most relaxed – the sound of ocean waves, rainfall, a fan? Find that sound and let it play for eight hours. Preferably use a battery-operated sound machine. Sleeping by a digital device that is on and connected to the internet can seriously disrupt sleep. Also, studies show that the health of your brain cells can be adversely affected.

Good sleep hygiene means training yourself to go to sleep. It takes practice. If you have poor habits or you work a night shift, it's harder. My husband worked rotating shifts for thirty years as a police officer. On a three-month rotation, he would work either days, evenings or graves, and it would take at least a week to get his body used to the next shift. When he worked grave-yard shifts, I would make the room absolutely dark by taping foil over the windows, like sleeping in a cave during the daytime in order to get his body to make enough melatonin. I used a lot of tricks to keep him as healthy as possible because I knew if he was going to be working shift work for so many years, then he would eventually have metabolic issues like diabetes.

Working nights is associated with higher risk of obesity, diabetes, heart disease, depression, anxiety and cancer. I didn't want that for my husband. So we spent 30 years working with his shift rotation without using sleep aids, just by changing his sleep environment.

What if you wake up in the middle of the night?

If you're having trouble staying asleep, remember that getting out of bed, checking your phone, turning on lights or doing anything outside of your bed reinforces awakeness. If you have to go to the bathroom, keep the lights off and do so with the least amount of stimulation. Then return to your cozy bed and go right back to sleep.

What if you can't go back to sleep? If this is the case, it's important to learn a relaxation technique to put yourself back to sleep. I recommend my go-back-to-sleep exercise, which I'll walk you through:

- First, be sure your pillow is in a good position and your pajamas and bed covers are comfortably situated. Lie flat on your back.

- Then, slowly contract your body one part at a time from your feet to your head. The key is to contract each part very consciously. All your attention should be telling that part of your body to contract and hold the contraction. First, contract your feet, then your lower legs, upper legs, buttocks, belly, back, chest, shoulders, arms, hands, neck, face, and squeeze your eyes shut. Hold the contraction of your entire body for 3 seconds.

- Very slowly relax one part at a time from your feet up to your head, and breathe.

- Repeat the contraction/relaxation wave twice.

If you are not able to reset your sleep cycles with these adult sleep training techniques in 14 days, then definitely consider supporting your hypothalamus nutraceutically.

Chapter 13

Adopt a Healing Mindset

Did you know that your emotional health affects your longevity? Yes, people with healing mindsets live healthier and longer than those with poor emotional health. A healing mindset reflects positive emotional and mental health.

A healing mindset takes some work - on your past traumas, inner child, codependent relationships and beliefs.

Your health and well-being reflects your beliefs. If you do not believe that you can heal, then there's not a perfect enough diet, enough activity, or enough sleep for you to reach optimal wellness. Your attitude towards your body, your health even yourself determines your sense of wellbeing.

You can believe yourself into illness and into wellness. Many years ago, I had a patient who I diagnosed with metastatic breast cancer. Unfortunately, she didn't have very long to live but she was worried about her niece who had become very concerned about her own breasts. So, my patient brought her fifteen-year-old niece to me for an evaluation.

I examined the girl and showed her how to examine her own breasts. Yet, as she watched her aunt suffer through breast cancer, this girl developed a mass too - in the same breast as her aunt.

As the child of her aunt's husband's sister, she was not even related to her aunt, nor was there a history of breast disease in her family. I believe her worry contributed to this young girl developing a breast mass. Fortunately, it ended up being a benign fibroadenoma.

When you worry about anything, it takes your mind away from the present.

Oftentimes, you're worried about the future or about what you've already done in the past. Truth is, your body very much responds to your present emotion and beliefs.

Your thoughts create your reality. Negative self-talk negatively affects your health and well-being. Every cell in your body is listening. Your hypothalamus is especially attuned to your emotions.

Just as a person rides a horse, your consciousness is the rider of your physical body.

Equestrians know that what they're thinking and feeling affects their mount as much if not more than what their hands and legs are doing. I've ridden horses since I was eleven years old and I've not found a horse I couldn't ride. I believe it's because I'm able to connect to the animal by staying present in my body and directing my thoughts and feelings towards what I wish the horse to do. If my mind is focused on what we're doing in the moment, my body naturally responds and the horse responds to my intentions. Your body responds to your mind much in the same way a horse responds to its rider.

Let me give you one more example of how your mind can affect your healing. In 2002, shortly after we moved to a new home, I had a riding accident. On a slick wet, foggy September morning, I took my mare on a trail ride. She was a high spirited animal, more go than whoa, but extremely athletic and sure footed on the single track trails. Yet, as we reached the top of the trail from which we had to go down a long paved street to loop back home, I had a vision of my mare going down. Knowing that thought creates reality, I quickly pushed that thought out of my mind. But sure enough, as we headed down the steep grade, my mare slipped on the wet pavement.

Luckily, I had envisioned it, so I was prepared and vaulted off and was not crushed under my horse. Unfortunately, I did hit my face on the street and knocked out my front teeth. I was able to find my teeth, catch my horse and get us back home. My husband took one look at me and drove me to the emergency dentist who said he couldn't save my teeth. I told the dentist that I believed he could. He rerooted my teeth, told me my teeth would die and sent me to the emergency room for x-rays. Thankfully, I did not have any broken bones. Still, I went home feeling sorry for myself. I was a mess and my bruised, swollen face was full of asphalt.

For about 24 hours I bemoaned my accident. I sat outside by the huge gaping hole in our backyard that we had dug for a swimming pool with my dogs surrounding me. Even my bruised horse came over and hung her head by me. I took a deep breath and centered myself and heard a voice.

This accident is a gift. It's time for you to learn how to heal yourself.

So I did what I had been telling my patients for years and got myself in the present moment. I became my own best cheerleader, cheerleading my body into healing. Every time I washed asphalt out of my skin, I told my body what a great job it was doing at healing. With every sip of liquid, since I couldn't eat anything solid, I told my body it was going to use those nutrients to heal.

I looked for what was working. I did not focus on my injuries. I coached myself into healing until my mindset was truly healing.

The accident happened on a Friday and on Sunday, we had friends over but they couldn't even tell anything had happened to me. By Monday, I went to go pick up my X rays and the emergency room staff didn't recognize me. My face was completely healed. And over 20 years later, my rerooted teeth are still alive and well.

You can heal anything with the right mindset.

Meditation, prayer, time to reflect – whatever you call it – health is not just physical. For optimal health, you must take care of your body, mind, and soul.

Meditation has been shown to lower stress hormones. It's great for hypertension, heart disease, and improves athletic performance. Your body needs you to connect to your soul.

The purpose of meditation is to quiet the mind. You don't have to sit still to meditate. You can take meditative walks. Swimming and sweeping can be meditative. Anything done with mindful repetition can be meditative.

When I first opened my integrative health clinic, I had a lot of spiritual gurus going through menopause seeking my care. What I mean by spiritual gurus is that they were highly adept psycho-spiritual healers. But physically, they needed help. At the time, I hadn't come out of the closet in terms of admitting my own intuitive healing abilities.

One I chose to barter with. We agreed; I would get her hormones balanced and she would teach me to meditate. Sitting before her cross-legged with my hands on my knees, thumbs touching forefingers in the ok sign, I closed my eyes and waited. She just laughed and said, "This is not your way. Go for a run with that black dog of yours." I hadn't told her about my animals but she was psychic.

So I took her advice and went on a run. Not a mile down the trail, my dog just stopped. She jumped onto a big boulder and stared down at me until I climbed up to join her and sat down.

Then she curled up against my back and I closed my eyes, took a few deep breaths, and a purple drop appeared and slowly flooded my consciousness. I was so enchanted by the purple drop that my mind stilled. Soon I was receiving answers to whatever was concerning me.

For years, I've found that being in nature brings me comfort and insight. It just takes a hike, run or swim to find that sweet spot to clear my mind and receive guidance. Now, it just takes intention.

One meditation I particularly love is more of a visualization. I use it to ground myself before doing healing work. A lot of healers, whether conventional or alternative, use their own energy to heal and eventually they get sick. Most healers have to work on taking care of themselves. I don't believe in using my own energy to heal others but tapping into the universal healing energies.

I begin by standing on the earth, preferably barefoot. But you can stand anywhere with shoes on as long as you're conscious of connecting to the earth. With my feet spaced as wide as my hips, I hold my hands down against my body, fingertips touching forming a V, arms relaxed and breathe mindfully.

This position makes me feel more open to receive, like my body is a chalice, ready to be filled up with light and wisdom.

I imagine the soles of my feet kissing the earth and the energy at the level of my hands near my root chakra to be a red glow. I drop that energy like roots down my legs through the soles of my feet and into the earth. I imagine those deep red roots sinking down through the crust of the earth and all the way to the center where I anchor myself.

I then allow the energy of the earth to flow back up through those roots and into my body. As the energy rises, it shifts from red to orange at my belly button and then golden yellow at the level of my diaphragm. I then take a deep breath and imagine that the crown of my head is opening like a camera aperture, allowing energy to flow in.

Violet energy pours into my crown chakra, turning indigo blue at the level of my third eye, then bright sky blue at the level of my throat.

Then I imagine the warm earth energies – red, orange, yellow – merge with the cool heavenly energies – violet, indigo, blue – in my heart. The deep forest green of my heart chakra blends with all the colors of the rainbow energies from heaven and earth. I allow the merged energy to flow from my heart to my hands.

Then I place my hands on whatever needs healing – a sore knee, a headache, a broken heart. I am an instrument of healing; it's not my energy but universal energy that does the healing. Plus, I'm never sucked dry when I tap into our beautiful healing earth and the multidimensional energies.

East meets West in your endocrine system

Energy affects matter. Your beliefs and thoughts are energy affecting the matter of your body. In the eastern philosophy of healing, treatments are focused on adjusting energy. Energy is more concentrated in seven points on your body - called chakras.

Like light waves, the chakras are identified by the color of the rainbow - red, orange, yellow, green, blue, indigo and purple.

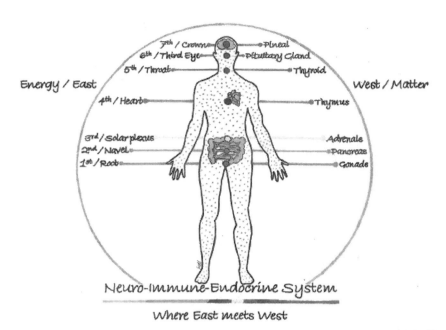

Energy / East   West / Matter

Neuro-Immune-Endocrine System

Where East meets West

Your seven chakras correspond to your seven endocrine glands. The root chakra correlates with your gonads, either ovaries or testes. The second chakra correlates with your pancreas. The third solar plexus chakra correlates with your adrenal glands. Your fourth heart chakra correlates with your thymus gland. Your fifth throat chakra is your thyroid. Your sixth third eye chakra is your pituitary gland. And your seventh crown chakra correlates with your pineal gland.

East meets west in your endocrine system. Your hormones allow energy to interface with matter. That's why it's so important to keep your hormones in harmony, and vitally important to optimize your hypothalamus function since it is the maestro of your symphony of hormonal messengers.

I find that focusing on my chakras with conscious breath helps me center myself. Honestly, I can't sit for long, yet when I meditate, I focus my consciousness on my endocrine glands. I envision the color of each chakra from root to crown and tune into my body. Even before I start clearing my mind, I tune into my body. Focusing on the matter and the energy of my body, chakra by chakra, helps to clear my mind. If I have any part of my body that's bothering me, I tune into that part to find out if it has any messages for me. For instance, when I've injured my legs, knees, ankles or feet, I often get the message that I need to slow down.

Tuning into my body and particularly my chakras where my endocrine glands lie is my way of meditating. Your way may be different. Perhaps you use prayer or yoga, certain music, light candles, be with nature to clear your mind, do some deep breathing and be with yourself or your higher power. Learning some form of meditation is important because it helps your mindset to shift into conscious healing. Without a healing mindset, it's difficult to heal your body.

Most of my patients have been sick for a long time and tend to have an ill mindset. They very much identify with their diseases. She's not Sue, she is diabetes. He's not Phil, he is Parkinson's. They identify with their disease rather than their truth. They often have trouble seeing beyond being their disease. They can't seem to envision themselves healthy.

A healing mindset starts with envisioning health and wellbeing. One way you can do that is by paying attention to what's working. So yes, I do tune into what's off, but I also scan my whole body for what's healthy and functioning well. And then I thank it. I'm in a place of gratitude for what's working. Your body responds to positive reinforcement. First, acknowledgement, then an expression of gratitude.

"Thank you, body! What a great job you're doing at healing."

Just like teaching a child and training an animal, positive reinforcement works tremendously well to train your body to do what you want it to do.

While your hypothalamus is the orchestrator of all of your symphony of neurotransmitters, immune factors and hormones, your mental attitude can actually change the way your hypothalamus is functioning. Your fear and worry handcuffs your hypothalamus. Your gratitude and positive affirmations help your hypothalamus to help you heal.

This mindset shift takes time, especially if you were raised in a family who looked at the negative side of life - the glass is half empty instead of the glass half full. It takes time to make that shift. I know it's possible because my husband was raised with a glass half empty attitude and definitely had a negative attitude when we got together.

It took a lot of years, but he definitely has shifted into more of a glass half full attitude. He tends to be much calmer, more accepting and ready to see the positive and not focus on the negative. Perhaps it's helped that he lives with a Pollyanna person like me, but I believe practicing being positive with our children and then with himself has made all the difference.

It does take time and practice. Part of the practice is surrounding yourself with people who are more positive, who have a more healing mindset. It's really hard to be in a healing mindset when everybody around you is yelling fire and running around like a chicken without a head. That's why people need groups of like-minded people to help them resonate towards health and well-being. We need healing circles.

Resonance means to attune to those around you. Energy is contagious. If you walk into a room where people are upset, angry, fearful, you can feel it. If you surround yourself with fearful people, you cannot help but be afraid. If you surround yourself with hopeful people, it's easier to be hopeful.

We need to be with people who have similar mindsets. So, if you're working on healing yourself, you need others who have healing mindsets, or at least are working on their mindsets. They become your cheerleaders and you coach each other through difficult situations. Everybody goes through stuff. Life is not easy, but coaching yourself through those situations can be challenging without a healing circle of positive people around you. Cheerleading each other can make a huge difference on your path to wellness.

I want to see you relaxed and comfortable in your body; healthy, with a clear mind, connected to the healing vibrations of those around you, to the earth itself. I find being in nature to be incredibly healing. We live surrounded by oaks in a neighborhood, appropriately named the Arbolada. Our small town is in an agriculture valley surrounded by mountains that the Native people - the Chumash - called the nest. It has a very healing energy and is a perfect place to do my healing work with patients and to create healing books and healing programs.

There is research that shows that being by trees and nature is very healing. In Japan, forest healing is prescribed where people are sent out to take walks in the forest to connect with nature and heal.

You need to find what works for you to get yourself into a healing mindset. Start by imagining what it would look like to be healthy and whole. What would life look like if you had all the energy you needed, if your hormones were in balance, and your brain was sharp, and you could sleep? What would life look like if you were optimally well?

Focusing on that positive image of yourself helps to draw you into that state of well-being. It's very much like how athletes perform. While being an athlete means physically working out and practicing their sport, it's also mental. A performance mindset means that the athlete imagines what is to happen and their body just does what it's trained to do. Their mind is not in their way.

Seeing in your mind's eye what life would be like when you're healthy and healed can actually shift you to that place. Yet, what happens when your brain pops up and says, "Oh my gosh, I got a pain. Oh, no, something bad is happening"? What can you do? You fix the language.

"Hello, pain. What are you trying to tell me? Am I going too fast and need to slow down a bit. Perhaps I didn't get enough sleep last night. It's okay. I hear you. What can I do to help myself heal?"

Then be your own cheerleader. I know that's hard, especially if you're not used to positive self-talk. That's why I created my Hormone Healing Circle. It started in 2017 when I gave an online course on hormone healing and presented it over 10 weeks. To give the participants some support, I formed an online community where we all met and supported each other. When the course was over, most of the people wanted to stay in the group. Where else can you find a compassionate community of like-minded people all working on healing their hormonal imbalances? In the resources section, I have more information on our Hormone Healing Circle.

Chapter 14

Nutraceutical Support for Your Hypothalamus

Your hypothalamus is dependent upon your nutritional status. Since it's not protected by the blood brain barrier, your hypothalamus receives micronutrients, amino acids and fatty acids from the bloodstream, utilizing these essential nutrients directly to orchestrate your symphony of hormones, neurotransmitters and immune factors.

Your hypothalamus needs specific nutrients for proper functioning, and a dysfunctional hypothalamus needs even more, which is why it can be difficult to get enough specific hypothalamic nutrition from your diet alone. That's where supplementation comes in.

Nutraceuticals designed to support your hypothalamus can help ensure your hypothalamus is functioning optimally. And that's important since your hypothalamus controls all of your body's vital functions, including digestion, detoxification, growth, repair, sleep, sex drive, reproduction, stress response, metabolism, body composition, immunity, weight, cognition, learning, memory and moods. Plus your hypothalamus controls what amino acids reach the brain to utilize for neurotransmitter production.

Research shows that hypothalamic neuronal health is very susceptible to nutrients. Without the proper micronutrients, your hypothalamus can become inflamed. Hypothalamic inflammation leads to the development and progression of diseases like obesity, insulin resistance, metabolic disorders as well as aging.

What nutrients does your hypothalamus need?

Amino acids

Your hypothalamus needs specific amino acids for proper functioning. Studies show that circulating amino acids affect hypothalamus performance and control of many functions. The amino acids your hypothalamus needs are the same amino acids that the rest of your body needs except in a different balance. Your hypothalamus is particularly sensitive to branched chain amino acids, but it needs all of the essential amino acids - those that your body cannot manufacture - and it needs extra doses of non-essential amino acids - those that your body can make - because often you don't get enough from your diet alone.

PUFAs

Your hypothalamus needs polyunsaturated fatty acids (PUFAs). Science has shown that the hypothalamus can grow and repair its own neuronal tissues with the help of PUFAs. Sea vegetation is rich in PUFAs as Omega-3 rich polyunsaturated fats make up a significant part of seaweed lipids. Green plant foods are also known to have a relatively high proportion of Omega-3 rich PUFAs.

Phytonutrients

Your hypothalamus utilizes plant-derived micronutrients to orchestrate its neuro-immune-endocrine functioning. Plant-based nutrients known as phytonutrients help modulate the communication between the hypothalamus, pituitary and lower endocrine glands like the HPA axis as well as the thyroid and gonadal axis. Hypothalamic phytonutrients come from herbs, sprouts and sea vegetation.

So, how can you get all of this vital hypothalamus nutrition - amino acids, PUFAs and phytonutrients? Even if your diet is pristine, it can be difficult. That's why I created a unique plant-based hypothalamus nutraceutical...

Genesis Gold®

You may remember from part one when I was working with some pretty hormonally challenged people who had issues with insomnia, anxiety, depression, thyroid disorders, and adrenal disorders. Most were overweight, all were fatigued and their sex hormones were out of balance. My research to try to figure out what was the root of their issue was how I rediscovered the hypothalamus.

What I didn't tell you was that once I found the root of the issue, I meditated to try to discover what to give my patients to heal hypothalamic dysfunction and maintain optimal wellness throughout their lifespan.

There are glandulars available - extracted from animals. Research on glandulars show that while they may be effective in the first few months, they don't maintain their efficacy. And that's because none of us were meant to eat glands from animals every day for the rest of our lives. Your liver treats those glands as a toxin after three to six months.

In the first few months, glandulars can be found in the glands they target. Adrenal glandular will be found in the adrenals, thyroid glandular in the thyroid and pituitary glandular in the pituitary gland. Yet, after three to six months, all glandulars ends up in the liver for detoxification.

Since your body has to eventually detoxify medicinal glandulars, and I was looking for long term hypothalamus support, I chose to avoid glandulars. Yet, I still couldn't find one product that would heal the hypothalamus and support optimal hypothalamic function long term. So, in order to help them detox and aid digestion, I had to give my patients multiple bottles of supplements to support their adrenals, thyroid, ovaries or testes, pituitary gland, cellular health, glucose metabolism, immune and brain function.

I had been studying particular amino acids important in the production of POMC - the hypothalamic mega pro hormone that orchestrates adrenal function, circadian rhythm, glucose metabolism and moods. Studies show that particular amino acids can actually change the way the hypothalamus functions. I was trying to figure this out when my intersex child, who was a teenager at this time, said, "Mom, quit struggling. Why don't you just meditate, then go to sleep and see what comes in your dreams?"

Always a prolific dreamer, I've dreamt everything important in my life. I dreamed of my husband before I met him. I dreamed of my children before they were even conceived, and they looked exactly like they did as young children. I dreamed of my integrative healthcare practice and the collaborating physician I would be working with well before opening Full Circle Family Health, and today, it's the longest running nurse practitioner led medical corporation in California. So I pay attention to my dreams.

That night, I did as my firstborn suggested. I meditated with the intention to know what I needed to feed my patients to heal their hypothalamus and upregulate their genetic expression, so they could enjoy optimal health — body, mind and soul.

I had the same dream every night for three months. In the dream, I was standing before the tree of life, holding a golden chalice. My sickest patients would come to me. We never spoke. I would offer them a drink from the chalice. When they did, I knew intuitively they were better. When I'd wake up in the morning, I would ask what was in the cup and just start writing. The first seven dreams revealed seven sets of amino acids.

Interestingly, these combinations of amino acids came to me as Aramaic letters. I didn't know they were Aramaic. I just wrote the symbols I saw in the dream upon awakening. I had a rabbi friend at the time, who was able to translate the symbols into specific Aramaic letters. Remember, amino acids are usually referred to by single letters. The first night's dream revealed the first set of seven amino acids - the same ones I had been studying which are related to POMC.

Over the next three months, a whole formula came to me in my dreams. I researched every single ingredient and many were similar to what I was already feeding my patients in multiple supplements. It was clear to me that the formula had to be consumed as a drink. In liquified form, the plant-based ingredients would be best absorbed and most active, most available to the hypothalamus.

Specific ratios of each amino acid were revealed in my dreams. I was working with an amino acid laboratory and was able to mix the seven sets of seven amino acids. I called the special hypothalamic amino acid blend Sacred Seven®.

Then I decided to see how it affected the hypothalamus. Over fifty of my patients volunteered to be part of my study group. Men, women and teens from 16 to 80 years of age took Sacred Seven® for six months. I hired a registered nurse to collect data - vital signs, bloodwork and questionnaires regarding how the subjects felt - at baseline, then monthly.

All subjects' symptoms of hypothalamic dysfunction improved - their blood-work took six months to show changes. One of the most remarkable findings was the shift in attitude for many of the subjects. They felt more attuned to their body's needs. Their dreams were more lucid. They made changes in their lives that improved their mental health and relationships.

It took me a few years to finally be able to manufacture the full hypothalamus support which I named Genesis Gold®. The Sacred Seven® hypothalamic amino acids are at the heart of the Genesis Gold® formula which is rich in Omega-3 PUFAs from sea vegetation, sprouted grains and legumes, as well as phytonutrient rich herbs and whole plant foods that specifically feed the hypothalamus to optimize its functioning.

Since 2003, Genesis Gold® has been available to my patients and I have had to do so much less to support their healing. Their hypothalamus function begins to optimize, they need much less hormonal support and the majority are able to get off of their medications. They finally get their lives back.

With Genesis Gold® optimizing hypothalamus function, they're able to sleep, get back into balance and manage stress better. Infertile patients become pregnant fairly easily. Honestly, I haven't had to do any infertility work since my patients began taking Genesis Gold®.

Now I know the hypothalamus can get what it needs to heal and maintain optimal function long term. I've had patients including myself who have been taking Genesis Gold® for over twenty years.

I believe that Genesis Gold® has enhanced our longevity, slowing down the aging process. After a long while, some people may forget why supporting their hypothalamus is important and stop taking Genesis Gold®. When they experience the aches and pains of aging, menstrual irregularities, poor sleep, digestive problems, they realize how much Genesis Gold® helps optimize hypothalamus function.

Yes, it's difficult to get everything you need from your diet alone. Plus we're constantly bombarded with toxins so your body needs so much more detoxification support. By taking Genesis Gold®, the majority of my patients are able to get off most of their other supplements.

Remember, your hypothalamus is not protected by the blood brain barrier. So, it is very receptive to the nutrients that are in Genesis Gold® - the amino acids, sea vegetation, sprouted plant foods, botanicals, adaptogenics and digestive aids. The plant-based nutrition in Genesis Gold® provides cellular, liver, and kidney detoxification support. The variety of botanicals helps improve cell membrane function, so your cells can utilize the nutrients in Genesis Gold® to help optimize receptor site function.

My patients who take Genesis Gold® consistently find that they need less bioidentical hormones and some eventually need no exogenous HRT as their endocrine glands start making their own hormones. Genesis Gold® is what my most challenging patient took, the one with panhypopituitaryism, who made none of her own hormones. By taking Genesis Gold®, she was able to get off all her exogenous hormones and her fertility was restored.

It does take time to heal your hypothalamus, at least 90 days. Why 90 days? Because that's the time it takes to rebalance the negative feedback system between the hypothalamus-pituitary and lower endocrine glands.

This is not a quick fix but a long term investment in your health. If you've been out of balance and hormonally challenged for many years, it'll take longer. After the first 90 days of hypothalamus support, it can take one month per year you've been out of balance to return to optimal health. That's why it took eighteen months for my patient with panhypopituitaryism to get off all of her hormones. Prior to taking Genesis Gold®, she had been out of balance for over 25 years.

Genesis Gold® Ingredients

Nutrient Group	Genesis Gold® Ingredients	What it does in your Body	Why its Important
Micronutrient Rich Blend of Whole Plant Foods from the Sea and the Land	Dulse/Bladderwrack, Blue-Green Algae, Chlorella, Spirulina, Kelp, Quinoa Sprouts , Hemp, Amaranth Sprouts, Broccoli Sprouts, Garbanzo Beans, Royal Jelly, Honey	Whole plant foods rich in phytonutrients provide protein, essential fatty acids, and fiber as well as activated vitamins, minerals and coenzymes to balance your diet and your pH	Phytonutrients naturally support your body's vital functions, reverse imbalances, optimize cellular energy production and detoxification and enhance healing.
Adaptogenic Herbal Blend	Ashwagandha, Astragalus, Banaba, Bayberry, Bilberry Leaf, Fo-ti, Ginkgo Biloba, Grape Seed, Green Tea, Hawthorne Berry, Licorice Root, Maitake Mushroom, Maca, Olive Leaf Extract, Pau d'arco, Pomegranate, Reishi Mushroom, Suma , Uña de Gato	Helps protect your body from stress, supports your immune system and balances your hormones	Your Hormones are the communication network of your body. If your hormones are out of balance, your body becomes sick and ages faster.
Detoxifying Phytonutrient Blend	Aloe Vera, Artichoke, Beet Root, Black Radish, Curcumin, Fennel, Flax Seed, Garlic, Ginger, Lemon Peel, Milk Thistle Seed	Helps your body rid itself of toxins through the liver, kidneys and colon	Your body functions best when it can clean itself of toxic waste from the environment
Plant Based Digestive Aides	Probiotics, Enzymes, Betaine HCL, Apple Cider Vinegar, Lecithin, Capsicum	Helps your body digest food and absorb essential nutrients	Proper digestion is crucial for your body to be able to absorb the nutrients necessary to heal and stay healthy
Sacred Seven® Amino Acids (plant derived)	Serine, Isoleucine, Asparagine, Cysteine, Threonine, Alanine, Valine, Proline, Ornithine, Histadine, Methionine, Tyrosine, Arginine, Aspartic acid, leucine, Glutamic Acid, Glutamine, Taurine, Glycine, Lysine, L-phenylalanine	By balancing the hypothalamus which is the maestro of the neurological, immune and endocrine system, your body's biochemistry functions at the highest level to help optimize your genetic potential	The only amino acid formula designed to support your Hypothalamus so it can keep your Hormones in Harmony® and optimize your Health

There are no hormones in Genesis Gold®, but it does improve receptor site activity. For instance, estrogen dominant women experience a balancing of their hormones and less estrogen activity.

All the hormonally challenged patients I presented in part two were started on hypothalamus support with Genesis Gold® and some utilized extra Sacred Seven® amino acids to hasten their healing. If my patients have food sensitivities or allergies to any of the plant ingredients in Genesis Gold®, they start on Sacred Seven® amino acids alone. After a few months, their sensitivities diminish and they can slowly add Genesis Gold®.

Since Genesis Gold® feeds you and your microbiome, those with intestinal dysbiosis, especially candida, start with Sacred Seven® until their gut microbiome can be rebalanced. Then, they can take Genesis Gold®. Sometimes I might suspect candida overgrowth or SIBO in a patient, but they want to get started on Genesis Gold® right away and not wait until we can get a stool analysis or breath test. If they experience gas and bloating shortly after taking Genesis Gold®, then we know their gut is out of balance and needs treatment.

Is Genesis Gold® all you need to optimize hypothalamus function?

Genesis Gold® supplies all the micronutrients necessary for optimal hypothalamus health. If you have other nutrient deficiencies, you may need particular vitamin, mineral or cofactor support until the deficiency is corrected. You still need to get the majority of your antioxidants from your diet.

For optimal hypothalamus health, you need nutraceutical support, enough sleep, exercise, proper nutrition and a healing mindset. Fortunately, with Genesis Gold®, it's easier to make the necessary lifestyle changes. Your body starts to demand the best food, sleep and activity for your body. Plus your attitude naturally shifts as your hypothalamus calms the stress response and balances your moods so it's easier to adopt a healing mindset.

I've had patients call Genesis Gold® - therapy in a bag. Their more lucid dreams helped them work through repressed issues and understand current life events at a deeper level. Psychotherapists have used Genesis Gold® with their clients to help them make needed breakthroughs.

When my husband first started taking Genesis Gold®, he didn't notice physical changes right away. Yet, as a police officer, he was under some considerable stress. His childhood security issues haunted him, so paying bills was not a pleasant affair. Whenever he got out his checkbook, the kids and the dogs left the room. Yet after a few months on Genesis Gold®, he was much more mellow.

Taking Genesis Gold® daily can help balance your hypothalamus and optimize its functioning, which helps balance your hormones and neurotransmitters and improve your immune function, digestion and detoxification. By providing your hypothalamus with the exact nutrients it needs for optimal functioning, Genesis Gold® can help balance moods, improve learning and memory, maintain proper weight and body composition, optimize glucose metabolism to reverse insulin resistance and improve hormonal function of the thyroid, adrenals, pituitary and gonads.

Supporting your hypothalamus with Genesis Gold® is a gift you give yourself for optimal health.

Part Four

For Healthcare Providers

Hypothalamus Dysfunction

For my colleagues who are healthcare providers, this part is for you.

Part one included anatomy and physiology of the hypothalamus, as well as etiology and pathophysiology of hypothalamus dysfunction.

Part two included six case studies with in depth pathophysiology of systems and diagnoses that are affected by hypothalamus dysfunction. Plus, I included therapeutic plans for each of the case studies.

Part three included the five pillars of optimizing hypothalamus function.

In part four, I will present hypothalamus dysfunction in a more systematic way for you to use as a quick reference.

Hypothalamus Dysfunction

Hypothalamus dysfunction is defined as insufficient production of hypo-thalamic hormones. Without adequate hypothalamus hormones, pituitary

Nuclei of the Hypothalamus

Anterior	Mid-Hypothalamus	Posterior
Preoptic Nucleus (PON) controls reproduction by producing gonadotropin releasing hormone (GnRH). The PON controls non-REM sleep and participates in thermoregulation.	**Arcuate Nucleus** (AN) produces growth hormone releasing hormone (GHRH), prolactin inhibiting hormone (PIH) which is dopamine and pro-opiomelanocortin (POMC). The AN is rich in leptin receptors and produces neuropeptide-Y (NPY). POMC controls adrenal function, circadian rhythm, glucose and fat metabolism and moods.	**Mammillary Nucleus** (MN) is connected to libido and controls memory, behavior and motivation.
Paraventricular Nucleus (PVN) produces oxytocin and some vasopressin. Oxytocin is the cuddle hormone helping to bond with others. The PVN produces thyroid releasing hormone to control thyroid function as well as cortico-releasing hormone to control adrenal cortisol production.	**Ventromedial Nucleus** (VMN) controls satiety, regulates glucose, and participates in thermogenesis or body heat production. The VMN is responsible for appetite, social and sexual behaviors.	**Posterior Hypothalamus Nucleus** (PHN) controls blood pressure, dilation of pupils, and thermoregulation to warm the body through shivering.
Supraoptic Nucleus (SON) primarily produces vasopressin and some oxytocin. Vasopressin is also known as antidiuretic hormone and controls salt water balance via the kidneys.	**Dorsimedial Nucleus** (DMN) is the emotional response center. The DMN controls blood pressure, heart rate, and stimulates gastrointestinal activity. The DMN produces prolactin releasing hormone (PRH). Prolactin helps regulate nocturnal immune function.	
Suprachiasmatic Nucleus (SCN) receives input from the retina to synchronize circadian rhythm. The SCN directs the pineal gland to produce melatonin.	**Lateral Hypothalamus Nucleus** (LHN) is responsible for wakefulness, orchestrating sleep and metabolism as well as feeding behaviors. The LHN also controls blood pressure, heart rate and water intake.	
Anterior Hypothalamus Nucleus (AHN) controls body temperature by regulating cooling - through vasodilation and sweating.		

function is diminished. Poor hypothalamus function affects all endocrine glands - thyroid, thymus, adrenals, ovaries, testes, pancreas, as well as the pineal gland.

Hypothalamus dysfunction affects brain function, immune function, digestion, metabolism and circadian rhythm. It also affects thermoregulation, appetite, energy, mood and memory. While the majority of hypothalamic dysfunction affects the HPA axis which influences adrenal function, all aspects of hypothalamus function can be affected.

The hypothalamus is composed of eleven nuclei that have different physiological functions. The main function of the hypothalamus is to maintain homeostasis by controlling endocrine and autonomic functions.

Through these eleven nuclei, the hypothalamus orchestrates all major body systems:

- Reproduction
- Metabolism
- Detoxification
- Blood pressure and heart rate
- Circadian rhythm
- Sleep and awareness
- Weight set point
- Food intake - hunger and satiety
- Glucose metabolism
- Fluid balance
- Temperature regulation
- Energy production

Hormones of the Hypothalamus

Name of Hypothalamic Hormone	Function
Gonatropin Releasing Hormone	GnRH stimulates the pituitary gland to make and secrete luteinizing hormone (LH) and follicle-stimulating hormone (FSH). FSH stimulates sperm production in men, while LH stimulates testosterone production. In women, FSH stimulates estrogen production and LH stimulates ovulation which results in progesterone production. GnRH also stimulates neurogenesis.
Growth Hormone Releasing Hormone	GHRH stimulates the pituitary to release growth hormone which stimulates growth in children, repair of tissues and impacts metabolism in adults.
Growth Inhibiting Hormone	GIH inhibits the release of growth hormone from the pituitary.
Prolactin Releasing Hormone	PRH stimulates the pituitary to release stored prolactin mainly at night to direct immune system modulation. Prolactin stimulates the secretion of other cytokines and the expression of cytokine receptors. Hyperprolactinemia is indicated in autoimmunity. Prolactin also deepens sleep.
Prolactin Inhibiting Hormone	PIH is dopamine. Dopamine is produced by the hypothalamus in abundance early in the day and shuts down the release of prolactin. Dopamine is the learning, memory and reward neurotransmitter.
Thyrotropin Releasing Hormone	TRH stimulates the release of thyroid stimulating hormone (TSH) from the pituitary in a negative feedback system with circulating thyroxine and triiodothyronine.
Cortico Releasing Hormone	CRH comes from POMC and stimulates the release of adrenocorticotropic hormone (ACTH) from the pituitary in a negative feedback system with circulating cortisol.
Lipotropin	Comes from POMC and promotes fat mobilization from adipose tissues, retaining excess amounts of fat in the liver and body. Lipotropin production follows ACTH - low at night and peaking in the morning.
Neuropeptide Y	NPY stimulates food intake particularly carbohydrates. While NPY is formed in the arcuate nucleus, it is active in the paraventricular, dorsomedial and ventromedial nuclei which regulate energy homeostasis. NPY regulates brain activity, resilience to stress, digestion, blood pressure, heart rate, body metabolism, and immune functions orexigenic.
Endorphins	β-endorphins are derived from POMC and induced by exercise and stress to block the sensation of pain, reduce stress and improve sense of wellbeing.
Melanocyte Stimulating Hormone	a-MSH comes from POMC and is considered the long route of adaptation. a-MSH regulates energy homeostasis and stimulates the secretion of ACTH, independent of CRH. MSH reduces fever, reduces inflammation, stimulates the formation of scar tissue, and suppresses appetite to conserve energy. β-MSH directly stimulates the pituitary production of ACTH and is inhibited by cortisol.
Oxytocin	Controls key aspects of the reproductive system, including childbirth and lactation, and aspects of human behavior - sexual arousal, recognition, trust, romantic attachment and mother–infant bonding. Oxytocin is known as the 'cuddle hormone".
Vasopressin	Also called antidiuretic hormone (ADH) regulates blood pressure, blood osmolality, and blood volume. Vasopressin is released mainly at night and acts to help regulate the circadian rhythm.
Orexin	Also called hypocretin is produced in the lateral hypothalamus and regulates arousal, wakefulness, and appetite.

- Immune function
- Autonomic nervous system
- Stress response
- Emotional expression
- Aggression
- Memory
- Moods
- Sexual arousal

Disorders of the hypothalamus may cause a variety of different signs and symptoms depending on the affected nuclei.

The hypothalamus produces thirteen master hormones that affect vital body systems.

Pathophysiology

If the hypothalamus is damaged by toxins, infections, malnutrition or injury, the endocrine system will be affected, including the hypothalamus-pituitary-adrenal axis, hypothalamus-pituitary-thyroid axis and hypothalamus-pituitary-gonadal axis.

Disorders that affect hypothalamic hormone secretion will affect pituitary hormone secretion. Neurosecretory hypothalamic hormones may also be affected. Hypothalamic control of immune function, metabolism and circadian rhythm may be affected.

Hypothalamic endoplasmic reticulum stress plays a critical role in mediating neuroinflammation and neuronal injury, as well as regulating food intake, energy expenditure and body weight.

Etiology

The causes of hypothalamus dysfunction are varied and include:

- Brain surgery
- Traumatic brain injury
- Brain tumors
- Radiation
- Chemotherapy
- Nutritional deficiencies (anorexia nervosa)
- Brain aneurysms
- Genetic disorders (Prader-Willi syndrome, Kallmann syndrome)
- Infections (EBV, SARS, TB, Lyme)
- Inflammatory disease (multiple sclerosis, neurosarcoidosis)
- Paraneoplastic syndromes
- Rapid-onset obesity (hypothalamic dysfunction, hypoventilation and autonomic dysregulation syndrome)
- Heat stroke
- Chronic stress

Epidemiology

Hypothalamic dysfunction, following traumatic brain injury, is reported in the range of 11-80%. Traumatic brain injury in children will triple their risk for developing central endocrine dysfunction compared to the general population. In children with hypothalamus dysfunction, girls have a 2:1 predominance. Hypothalamus dysfunction accounts for 20 to 35% of the cases of secondary amenorrhea in the United States. Pediatric cancer survivors have a prevalence of over 40% for hypothalamic-pituitary dysfunction, predominantly for growth hormone.

Subjective Assessment

Signs and symptoms of hypothalamic dysfunction are varied according to what part of the hypothalamus is damaged, including:

- Sympathetic or parasympathetic complaints
- Fatigue
- Temperature dysregulation - hypothermia, hot flashes, night sweats, fevers
- Appetite changes - anorexia or hyperphagia
- Weight loss or weight gain, with or without changes in appetite
- Sleep disorders - trouble initiating sleep or staying asleep
- Pain - especially trigger point tenderness
- Mood disorders - anxiety , depression
- Libido issues
- High blood pressure or low blood pressure
- Water retention
- Dehydration
- Excessive thirst
- Excessive urination
- Irritable bowel with maldigestion, malabsorption, constipation, diarrhea
- Amenorrhea
- Irregular periods
- Infertility

- Osteoporosis
- Delayed puberty
- Sarcopenia
- Weakness
- Premature aging
- Lack of motivation
- Inability to bond with others
- Maladaptive stress response
- Skin rashes, acne and eczema

To help elicit clues to hypothalamus dysfunction, ask patients about:

- When symptoms began
- Progression of symptoms
- Major or chronic stressors
- Head injuries
- Infections - Epstein Barr virus, tuberculosis, lymes and/or SARS-coV-19
- Diagnoses of myalgic encephalomyelitis/chronic fatigue syndrome or fibromyalgia
- Childhood health
- Adverse Childhood Events
- Toxic exposures to heavy metals, pesticides, herbicides, chemotherapy
- Weight history
- Dietary history
- Female gynecological history

- Male reproductive, sexual history
- Family history of genetic disorders

Objective Assessment

Since the signs and symptoms of hypothalamic dysfunction can be non-specific, the history and physical examination of patients must be tailored according to the patient's clinical manifestation.

Physical exam should include:

- Body habitus
- Distribution of body fat - apple shaped (cortisol driven/insulin resistant) pear shaped (estrogen dominance)
- Distribution of muscle - sarcopenia (flat posterior deltoids /androgen deficiency)
- Skin - signs of aging, melasma acanthosis nigricans, loss of pigment (vitiligo or small depigmented spots on extremities indicates estrogen deficiency) , any rashes or acne
- Hair distribution - loss of pubic hair (low adrenal androgens), loss of body hair, thinning eyebrows, loss of outer third of eyebrows (low thyroid), hirsutism or male pattern hair on a female (high androgens), loss of head hair (diffuse - low estrogen/low thyroid vs thinning at temples and crown - high androgens)
- Cardiovascular - heart rate and rhythm, carotid bruits, pulses , edema
- Breast exam both male and female checking for masses and nipple discharge
- Abdomen - hepatosplenomegaly, abdominal masses or tenderness
- Thyroid - size, shape, nodularity, tenderness (if enlarged may indicate autoimmune thyroiditis)

- Female pelvic exam - uterine fibroids, ovarian masses

- Male genital exam - inguinal hernias, testicular size and masses

- Rectal exam - if over 40 - checking for masses and occult blood, and in men, checking size and texture of prostate.

Labs

Diagnostic workup for hypothalamic dysfunction depends on the patient's clinical condition, signs and symptoms. Typical workup, includes blood and urine laboratory tests such as:

Chemistry panel to check electrolytes as well as liver and kidney health.

HGBA1C to evaluate insulin sensitivity.

Advanced lipid panel with subparticle sizes and lipoproteins. Steroid hormones are created from large particle low density lipids (LDL). Lipoprotein A reflects small density LDL and if elevated, might indicate an increased risk of arteriosclerosis, and potential decrease in vascular perfusion to the hypothalamus.

CRP-hs may be elevated in cases of hypothalamic micro inflammation.

Vitamin D - a vital prohormone acts to improve cell receptor site function.

Thyroid panel looking at the ratio of TSH to fT4 and fT3. If TSH is low normal in the face of low normal active thyroid hormones or vice versa, if TSH is high normal with high normal fT_4 and fT_3 levels, then there is a miscommunication at the hypothalamic-pituitary-thyroid axis - a sign of hypothalamus dysfunction. Add reverse T_3 if suspect metabolic issues as reflected by high body fat percentage or fatigue.

Thyroid autoantibodies - if suspect autoimmune thyroiditis, include thyroid peroxidase antibodies (TPO), thyroglobulin antibodies (TBGab) or thyroid stimulating immunoglobulin (TSI), which reflects autoimmune hyperthyroiditis.

DHEA-S - DHEA production follows cortisol production but unlike cortisol, DHEA-S can be measured anytime of the day, and is not immediately reflective of acute stress. If DHEA-S levels are out of range, then order an unconjugated DHEA to measure adrenal reserve and pregnenolone - a precursor hormone to adrenal androgens.

Cortisol - If out of normal limits at 8am, check hypothalamus-pituitary-adrenal axis by ordering fasting 8am ACTH with serum cortisol.

FSH - drawn day 3-5 of menstrual cycle or anytime if amenorrheic or menopausal - reflects female estrogen adequacy.

LH - reflects ovarian progesterone production in women or testicular testosterone production in men.

Progesterone measured in infertile women during mid luteal phase to determine ovulation and if adequate progesterone to carry through first trimester until placenta can produce progesterone.

Testosterone and free testosterone in males. If free testosterone is low, sex hormone binding globulin (SHBG) is probably elevated. Order DHT (dihydrotestosterone) in males and hirsute females.

Prolactin drawn between 8-9 AM, there must be no nipple stimulation at least 24 hours prior.

IgF-1 reflects human growth hormone (HGH) activity.

ANA quantitative - if elevated order specific antibody testing based on titer and pattern.

HCP Labs to help determine Hypothalamus Dysfunction

Lab	Reference Values	Indication	Best Measured
HGBA1C	4.0-5.6% 5.7 -6.1% >6.1 %	normal indicates insulin resistance indicates diabetes	
C-Peptide	0.5 to 2.0 ng/mL		
Fasting Lipid Panel with subparticle sizes			
hs-CRP	<1mg/l	elevation indicates cardiovascular inflammation	
25-hydroxyl Vitamin D	40-50ng/ml	optimal	
TSH	0.5 to 5.0 mIU/L		
fT4	0.7 to 1.9ng/dL		
fT3	2.3 – 4.1 pg/mL		
Thyroid autoantibodies – TPO, TGBab, TSI		order if suspect auto immune thyroiditis	
DHEA-S	Typical normal ranges for females are: • Ages 18 to 19: 145 to 395 µg/dL • Ages 20 to 29: 65 to 380 µg/dL • Ages 30 to 39: 45 to 270 µg/dL • Ages 40 to 49: 32 to 240 µg/dL • Ages 50 to 59: 26 to 200 µg/dL • Ages 60 to 69: 13 to 130 µg/dL • Ages 69 and older: 17 to 90 µg/dL Typical normal ranges for males are: • Ages 18 to 19: 108 to 441 µg/dL • Ages 20 to 29: 280 to 640 µg/dL • Ages 30 to 39: 120 to 520 µg/dL • Ages 40 to 49: 95 to 530 µg/dL • Ages 50 to 59: 70 to 310 µg/dL • Ages 60 to 69: 42 to 290 µg/dL • Ages 69 and older: 28 to 175 µg/dL		
unconjugated DHEA	18-40 years 1330-7780 ng/L 40-67 years 630-4700 ng/L,		
Cortisol	5 to 25 mcg/dL		if indicated draw at 6 am
ACTH	10 to 60 pg/mL with cortisol	if cortisol is abnormal	draw 8am
Pregnenolone	Men: 10 to 200 ng/dL Women: 10 to 230 ng/dL Children: 10 to 48 ng/dL	draw if DHEA low	
FSH	Women: 1.5 to 12.4 mIU/mL		on day 3-5 of menstrual cycle (day 1 is the first day you bleed),1.5 to 12.4 mIU/mL, drawn anytime if you're not menstruating
Testosterone	Men: 300 to 1,000 nanograms ng/dL free testosterone: 4.5-25.0 ng/dl dihydrotestosterone: 14 to 77 ng/dL		
LH	Men: 1.24 to 7.8 IU/mL Women, follicular phase of menstrual cycle: 1.68 to 15 IU/mL Women, midcycle peak: 21.9 to 56.6 IU/mL	if suspect menopause, premature ovarian failure, or hypogonadism in men	
Progesterone	5 to 20 ng/mL		in infertile women – drawn mid luteal phase (about 7 days before expected period)
SHBG	Males: 10 to 57 nmol/L Females (nonpregnant): 18 to 144 nmol/L		
Prolactin	ideally under 9 ng /ml at that time • Men: less than 20 ng/mL, • Women: less than 25 ng/mL, • Pregnant women: 80 to 400 ng/mL		must be drawn 8-9am

IGF-1	Males: • 0-11 months 16-356 ng/mL • 1 year 14-258 ng/mL • 2 years 16-222 ng/mL • 3 years 23-229 ng/mL • 4 years 30-238 ng/mL • 5 years 37-250 ng/mL • 6 years 47-279 ng/mL • 7 years 54-312 ng/mL • 8 years 61-356 ng/mL • 9 years 67-405 ng/mL • 10 years 73-456 ng/mL • 11 years 79-500 ng/mL • 12 years 84-551 ng/mL • 13 years 90-589 ng/mL • 14 years 95-638 ng/mL • 15 years 99-688 ng/mL • 16 years 104-658 ng/mL • 17 years 107-615 ng/mL • 18-22 years 91-442 ng/mL • 23-25 years 66-342 ng/mL • 26-30 years 60-329 ng/mL • 31-35 years 54-310 ng/mL • 36-40 years 48-292 ng/mL • 41-45 years 44-275 ng/mL • 46-50 years 40-259 ng/mL • 51-55 years 37-248 ng/mL • 56-60 years 34-242 ng/mL • 61-65 years 35-220 ng/mL • 66-70 years 32-205 ng/mL • 71-75 years 32-200 ng/mL • 76-80 years 33-192 ng/mL • 81-85 years 28-185 ng/mL • 86-90 years 33-179 ng/mL • > or =91 years 32-073 ng/mL Tanner Stage reference ranges: Males: • Stage I: 45-253 ng/mL • Stage II: 106-482 ng/mL • Stage III: 245-511 ng/mL • Stage IV: 225-578 ng/mL • Stage V: 227-546 ng/mL	Females: • 0-11 months 14-492 ng/mL • 1 year 23-245 ng/mL • 2 years 28-256 ng/mL • 3 years 31-249 ng/mL • 4 years 35-257 ng/mL • 5 years 38-284 ng/mL • 6 years 39-246 ng/mL • 7 years 44-279 ng/mL • 8 years 51-364 ng/mL • 9 years 61-408 ng/mL • 10 years 71-495 ng/mL • 11 years 88-545 ng/mL • 12 years 104-645 ng/mL • 13 years 120-719 ng/mL • 14 years 150-729 ng/mL • 15 years 147-691 ng/mL • 16 years 133-671 ng/mL • 17 years 149-509 ng/mL • 18-22 years 85-570 ng/mL • 23-25 years 75-329 ng/mL • 26-30 years 66-305 ng/mL • 31-35 years 59-279 ng/mL • 36-40 years 54-258 ng/mL • 41-45 years 49-243 ng/mL • 46-50 years 44-221 ng/mL • 51-55 years 40-217 ng/mL • 56-60 years 37-208 ng/mL • 61-65 years 35-204 ng/mL • 66-70 years 34-194 ng/mL • 71-75 years 34-187 ng/mL • 76-82 years 34-182 ng/mL • 81-85 years 34-177 ng/mL • 86-90 years 33-175 ng/mL • > or =91 years 25-175 ng/mL Females: • Stage I: 86-925 ng/mL • Stage II: 118-451 ng/mL • Stage III: 258-529 ng/mL • Stage IV: 224-986 ng/mL • Stage V: 188-512 ng/mL	to determine HGH activity	
ANA	1:40 serum dilution		>1.320 suspect autoimmunity and run reflex antibodies	

Other diagnostic tests may include:

- Blood and urine osmolality - if suspect issues with vasopressin (ADH)
- Genetic analysis if suspect Kallman or Prader-Willis
- Visual field test - if suspect a hypothalamic-pituitary tumor
- Brain imaging: magnetic resonance imaging (gold standard) or computed tomographic scan (for emergency cases)

Simple trifecta of hypothalamic function is comparing thyroid panel, DHEA-S and HGBA1C together. These lower endocrine markers reflect hypothalamic POMC function. If out of range with one another, suspect hypothalamus dysfunction.

Once the diagnosis of hypothalamic dysfunction is made, treatment varies according to the individual needs of the patient. No two cases are exactly the same. Some patients need full hormone supplementation, others need partial supplementation, most need to make lifestyle modifications and will need nutraceutical hypothalamus support.

Differential Diagnosis

Sometimes, it is difficult to differentiate between pituitary and hypothalamic dysfunction. Depending on the patient's condition, certain diseases can mimic the signs and symptoms of hypothalamic dysfunction.

In hormonal deficiencies, the differential diagnosis, includes pituitary gland lesions as well as the target organ involved (central hypothyroidism due to hypothalamic or anterior pituitary dysfunction vs. thyroid gland dysfunction).

In electrolyte imbalances, such as hypernatremia due to diabetes insipidus causes include central diabetes insipidus (due to lack of ADH production and secretion by the hypothalamus) vs. nephrogenic diabetes insipidus (due to ADH resistance or ADH receptor malfunction in the collecting duct of the kidneys).

Increased appetite can result from genetic abnormalities that cause hypothalamic dysfunction as seen in Prader-Willi syndrome, or can be due to other conditions such as hyperthyroidism.

Sleep disorders may be caused by a deficiency in hypothalamic hormones such as melanocyte stimulating hormone. Substance use, stimulants that alter sleep, psychiatric conditions, such as generalized anxiety disorder or major depressive disorder and REM-sleep behavior disorders can also affect sleep patterns.

Hypothalamus dysfunction plays a role in other health issues

Acromegaly and pituitary gigantism: Rare disorders of growth due to excessive release of growth hormone from the pituitary gland which is controlled by hypothalamus.

Addictions: Hypothalamus is often at the root of addictive behaviors. Cocaine addiction has recently been associated with hypothalamic dysfunction.

Aging: Hypothalamus micro inflammation initiates cellular aging. Hypothalamic micro inflammation can arise under nutritional conditions, leading to metabolic syndrome.

Amenorrhea: The absence of a period for more than three months in people assigned female at birth (AFAB), who previously had regular periods or more than six months in people AFAB, who have irregular menstruation. The most common cause of amenorrhea is hypothalamic dysfunction.

Autoimmunity: The hypothalamus regulates immune function. Studies show that hypothalamus dysfunction is often at the root of autoimmune conditions.

Cardiovascular disease: Patients with hypothalamic-pituitary disease are known to have increased cardiovascular risk.

Central hypothyroidism: A rare disorder that occurs due to both hypothalamic and pituitary disorders. The most common cause is a pituitary tumor such as a pituitary adenoma.

Central Obesity: Studies have shown that obese people with thyroid symptoms often have hypothalamic dysfunction. Dysfunctional insulin and leptin receptors within the hypothalamus may have a role in hypothalamic obesity. Diets with abundant saturated fatty acids cause mitochondrial dysfunction and inflammatory response in the hypothalamus, producing hypothalamic dysfunction, which promotes obesity. Activation of hypothalamic inflammatory pathways results in the uncoupling of caloric intake and energy expenditure, fostering overeating and further weight gain.

CFS/Myalgic Encephalitis: The hypothalamus controls mitochondrial energy output and cellular metabolism. Hypothalamus dysfunction is often at the root of chronic fatigue syndrome/myalgic encephalitis.

Diabetes insipidus: Hypothalamus dysfunction interferes with production and release of vasopressin, causing hyper renal function.

Diabetes/insulin resistance: Hypothalamic inflammation links central insulin resistance to diabetes. Hypothalamic regulation of feeding, body weight and glucose homeostasis is mediated by multiple signaling pathways, including insulin signaling.

Hyperprolactinemia: A decrease in hypothalamic dopamine levels causes an increase in prolactin levels. Causes may include a pituitary adenoma or damage to hypothalamic neurons.

Hypothalamic-pituitary disorders: Because of the close interactions between the hypothalamus and pituitary gland, conditions that affect either are often caused by hypothalamus dysfunction.

Hypopituitarism: The pituitary gland does not make enough stimulating hormones or its own hormones. Damage to the hypothalamus can cause hypopituitarism.

Insomnia: The hypothalamus controls circadian rhythm and is at the root of most sleep disorders, including sleep apnea.

Kallmann syndrome: Has a genetic link to hypothalamic disease, causing such hypothalamic problems in children as delayed or no puberty.

Mood disorders: Studies have shown that the hypothalamus is 5% smaller in people with clinical depression and bipolar condition.

Pain: Studies show that the hypothalamus regulates pain sensation and hypothalamus dysfunction is often at the root of chronic pain disorders like fibromyalgia.

Prader-Willi syndrome: An inherited disorder which causes the hypothalamus not to recognize satiation, resulting in hyperphagia and morbid obesity.

Reproductive issues/Infertility: The hypothalamus regulates reproduction, including the timing of puberty, menstrual periods, fertility, menopause and andropause.

Syndrome of inappropriate antidiuretic hormone: Elevated hypothalamic antidiuretic hormone level can be caused by stroke, hemorrhage, infection, trauma, cancer and certain medications.

Prognosis

Prognosis depends on the patient's resulting condition. Many of the manifestations caused by hypothalamic dysfunctions are treatable, in particular, hormone deficiency or overproduction. In patients with a hormone deficiency, hormone replacement therapy is the primary treatment.

Addressing hypothalamus dysfunction with nutraceutical support and lifestyle management may help improve hypothalamus-pituitary axis communication.

Complications

Hormonal deficiencies, such as low production of TRH or CRH, can cause central hypothyroidism or adrenal insufficiency, respectively. These may result in systemic complications such as cardiac issues and elevated cholesterol in the case of central hypothyroidism and low blood pressure and electrolyte disturbances in the setting of adrenal insufficiency.

Complications of insufficient production of GHRH include weakness, short stature, osteoporosis and high cholesterol. Pituitary sex hormones and oxytocin deficiencies will produce complications or infertility, erectile dysfunction, breastfeeding problems, labor difficulty, osteoporosis and decreased sexual stimulation and response.

For structural causes of hypothalamic dysfunction, as seen in patients with brain tumors, the complications associated are elevated intracranial pressure, seizures, blindness or visual field defects.

Assessment

Hypothalamus Dysfunction ICD-10-CM E23.3

Plan

Treatment depends on the etiology of the hypothalamic dysfunction, as well as the patient's presenting signs and symptoms.

For hormonal deficiencies, therapeutic hormone replacement is used. Kallmann syndrome requires lifelong sex hormone replacement.

For tumors, surgery or radiation may be required. Hypothalamic gliomas are usually observed. A biopsy can be performed for those not involving the optic chiasm and tracts. For hypothalamic hamartomas, if symptomatic with uncontrolled seizures, surgery, thermoablation or radiosurgery is recommended.

Nutritional guidance and appetite suppressants may be used to regulate the patient's appetite.

Delayed puberty in Frohlich syndrome is treated in females with estrogen and later estrogen-progesterone; in males with human chorionic gonadotropin and later with testosterone.

Therapeutic plans may include:

- Hypothalamus nutraceutical protocol
- Nutritional plan
- Activity/exercise plan
- Sleep plan
- Stress reduction plan - psychosocial support

More support for managing hypothalamus dysfunction can be found at https://genesisgold.com/hypothalamus/

References

PART ONE

Is human obesity an inflammatory disease of the hypothalamus? Sonnefeld, L., Rohmann, N., Geisler, C., & Laudes, M.; European Journal of Endocrinology; 2023.

Dysfunction of the hypothalamic-pituitary-adrenal axis in critical illness: A narrative review for emergency physicians; Lucas Oliveira Marino and Heraldo Possolo Souza; European Journal of Emergency Medicine; 2020; 27(6): 406–413.

Molecular Mechanisms of Hypothalamic Insulin Resistance; Hiraku Ono; International Journal of Molecular Sciences; 2019; 20(6): 1317.

Inhibition of Hypothalamic Inflammation Reverses Diet-Induced Insulin Resistance in the Liver; Marciane Milanski; Ana P. Arruda; Andressa Coope; Letícia M. Ignacio-Souza; Carla E. Nunez; Erika A. Roman; Talita

Romanatto; Livia B. Pascoal; Andrea M. Caricilli; Marcio A. Torsoni; Patricia O. Prada; Mario J. Saad; Licio A. Velloso; Obesity Studies; 2012; vol 61; issue 6.

New Insights into the Role of Insulin and Hypothalamic-Pituitary-Adrenal (HPA) Axis in the Metabolic Syndrome; Joseph A. M. J. L. Janssen; International Journal of Molecular Sciences; 2022, 23(15), 8178.

"Hypothalamic Microinflammation" Paradigm in Aging and Metabolic Diseases

Dongsheng Cai and Sinan Khor; Journal of Cell Metabolism; 2019.

Hypothalamic dysfunction in obesity; Lynda M. Williams; Proceedings of the Nutrition Society; 2012; 71, 521–533.

Cardiovascular disease, hypertension, dyslipidaemia and obesity in patients with hypothalamic-pituitary disease; D Deepak, N J Furlong, J P H Wilding, and I A MacFarlane; Postgraduate Medical Journal; 2007; 83(978): 277–280.

Hypothalamic dysfunction in heart failure; Antonios Rigas, Dimitrios Farmakis, Georgios Papingiotis, Georgios Bakosis, John Parissis; Heart Failure Reviews; 2018; 23(1).

One Step from Prediabetes to Diabetes: Hypothalamic Inflammation? Dongsheng Cai; Endocrinology; 2012; 153(3): 1010–1013.

The impact of antidiabetic treatment on human hypothalamic infundibular neurons and microglia; Martin J.T. Kalsbeek, Samantha E.C. Wolff, Nikita L. Korpel,Susanne E. la Fleur, Johannes A. Romijn, Eric Fliers, Andries Kalsbeek, Dick F. Swaab, Inge Huitinga, Elly M. Hol, and Chun-Xia Yi; JCI Insight. 2020; 5(16): e133868.

Prolactin and Autoimmunity; Vânia Vieira Borba, Gisele Zandman-Goddard, and Yehuda Shoenfeld; Frontier Immunology. 2018; 9:73.

Maternal obesity causes fetal hypothalamic insulin resistance and disrupts development of hypothalamic feeding pathways; L Dearden, S Buller, I C Furigo, D S Fernandez-Twinn, S E Ozanne; Molecular Metabolism; 2020; 42:101079.

Endoplasmic Reticulum Stress Coping Mechanisms and Lifespan Regulation in Health and Diseases; Sarah R Chadwick, Patrick Lajoie; Frontiers in Cell Developmental Biology; 2019; 7:84.

The role of hypothalamic endoplasmic reticulum stress in schizophrenia and antipsychotic-induced weight gain: A narrative review; Ruqin Zhou, Meng He, Jun Fan, Ruoxi Li, Yufeng Zuo, Benben Li, Guanbin Gao, Taolei Sun; Frontiers in Neuroscience; 2022;16:947295.

Maternal obesity-induced endoplasmic reticulum stress causes metabolic alterations and abnormal hypothalamic development in the offspring; Soyoung Park, Alice Jang, Sebastien G Bouret; PLoS Biol; 2020; 18(3): e3000296.

Metabolic syndrome as a common comorbidity in adults with hypothalamic dysfunction; Zhuoran Xu et al; Frontiers in Endocrinology; 2022; Volume .

Ischemic and oxidative damage to the hypothalamus may be responsible for heat stroke; Sheng-Hsien Chen, Mao-Tsun Lin, Ching-Ping Chang; Current Neuropharmacology; 2013; 11(2):129-40.

Why obese patients may have normal thyroid tests despite 'thyroid symptoms'" Sakkal S, et al; American Association of Clinical Endocrinologists 2014; 1974326.

Hypothyroidism and obesity: An intriguing link; Debmalya Sanyal, Moutusi Raychaudhuri, Indian Journal of Endocrinology Metabolism; 2016; 20(4): 554–557.

Hypothalamic Control of Systemic Glucose Homeostasis: The Pancreas Connection; Macarena Pozo, Marc Claret; Trends in Endocrinology and Metabolism; 2018; Volume 28, issue 8.

The Brain–to–Pancreatic Islet Neuronal Map Reveals Differential Glucose Regulation From Distinct Hypothalamic Regions; Wilfredo Rosario, Inderroop Singh, Arnaud Wautlet, Christa Patterson, Jonathan Flak, Thomas C. Becker, Almas Ali, Natalia Tamarina, Louis H. Philipson, Lynn W. Enquist, Martin G. Myers, Jr., Christopher J. Rhodes; Diabetes; 2016

Hypothalamic control of thymic function; K Hirokawa, M Utsuyama, S Kobayashi; Cellular Molecular Biology; 2001.

Role of prolactin and growth hormone on thymus physiology; V De Mello-Coelho, W Savino, M C Postel-Vinay, M Dardenne; Developmental Immunology; 1998; 6(3-4):317-23.

Effects of GnRH immunization on the reproductive axis and thymulin; Shiping Su, Xiaoxia Sun, Xiuhong Zhou, Fuigui Fang, Yunsheng Li; Endocrinology; 2015; 226(2):93-102.

Physiology of GnRH and Gonadotropin Secretion; Pedro Marques, Karolina Skorupskaite, Kavitha S. Rozario, Richard A. Anderson, Jyothis T. George; Endotext; 2022.

Oxytocin and social functioning; Candace Jones,et al;Dialogues Clinical Neuroscience; 2017; 19(2): 193–201.

A novel role of oxytocin: Oxytocin-induced well-being in humans; Etsuro Ito,Rei Shima, Tohru Yoshioka; Biophysics and Physicobiology; 2019; 16: 132–139.

Relationship between the pineal body and the hypothalamo-hypophyseal system. V. Melatonin inhibition of the gonadotropic activity of the hypothalamo-hypophyseal system; E A Siutkin, O G Krivosheev, N A Nabatchikova, V A Isachenkov; 1980; 26(2):53-7.

Pineal-dependent increase of hypothalamic neurogenesis contributes to the timing of seasonal reproduction in sheep; Martine Batailler, Didier Chesneau, Laura Derouet, Lucile Butruille, Stéphanie Segura, Juliette Cognié, Joëlle Dupont, Delphine Pillon, Martine Migaud; Scientific Reports; 2018; volume 8, Article number: 6188.

Physiology of the Pineal Gland and Melatonin; Josephine Arendt, PhD, Anna Aulinas, MD, PhD.: Endotext; 2022.

Neural basis for regulation of vasopressin secretion by anticipated disturbances in osmolality; Angela Kim, Joseph C Madara, Chen Wu, Mark L Andermann, Bradford B Lowell; Elife; 2021; 10: e66609.

60 YEARS OF POMC: Lipotropin and beta-endorphin: a perspective; D G Smyth; Journal of Molecular Endocrinology; 2016; 56(4): T13-25.

Brain regulation of appetite and satiety; Rexford S. Ahima, MD, PhD, Daniel A. Antwi, PhD; Endocrinology Metabolism Clinical North America. 2008; 37(4): 811–823.

Sleep and Metabolism: Implication of Lateral Hypothalamic Neurons; Lukas T Oesch, Antoine R Adamantidi; Frontiers in Neurological Neuroscience; 2021;45:75-90.

The Arcuate Nucleus of the Hypothalamus and Metabolic Regulation: An Emerging Role for Renin–Angiotensin Pathways; Darren Mehay, Yuval Silberman, and Amy C. Arnol; International Journal of Molecular Science; 2021; 22(13): 7050.

Insulin synthesized in the paraventricular nucleus of the hypothalamus regulates pituitary growth hormone production; Jaemeun Lee, Kyungchan Kim, Jae Hyun Cho, Jin Young Bae, Timothy P O'Leary, James D Johnson, Yong Chul Bae, Eun-Kyoung Kim; Journal of Clinical Investigation; 2020; 5(16):e135412.

Hypothalamic regulation of pancreatic secretion is mediated by central cholinergic pathways in the rat; Ying Li, Xiaoyin Wu, Jinxia Zhu, Jin Yan, Chung Owyang; Journal of Physiology; 2003; 552(Pt 2): 571–587.

Neuropeptide Y in normal eating and in genetic and dietary-induced obesity; B Beck; Philos Trans R Soc London Biological Sciences; 2006; 361(1471): 1159–1185.

A gut-brain axis mediates sodium appetite via gastrointestinal peptide regulation on a medulla-hypothalamic circuit; Jo-An Wei et al; Science Advances; 2023; Vol 9, Issue 7.

Dysfunction of the hypothalamic-pituitary adrenal axis and its influence on aging: the role of the hypothalamus; Melanie Spindler, Marco Palombo, Christiane M. Thiel; Scientific Reports; 2023; volume 13, Article number: 6866.

PART TWO

The interplay between thyroid and liver: Implications for clinical practice; E Piantanida, S Ippolito, D Gallo, E Masiello, P Premoli, C Cusini, S Rosetti

, J Sabatino , S Segato , F Trimarchi , L Bartalena , M L Tanda; Journal of Endocrinology Investigations; 2020; 43(7):885-899.

The Underlying Mechanisms: How Hypothyroidism Affects the Formation of Common Bile Duct Stones—A Review; Johanna Laukkarinen, Juhani Sand, Isto Nordback; Hepato-Pancreatico-Biliary Surgery; 2012; 102825.

Thyroid-stimulating hormone regulates hepatic bile acid homeostasis via SREBP-2/HNF-4α/CYP7A1 axis; Yongfeng Song Chao Xu Shanshan Shao   Jun Liu   Wanjia Xing, Jin Xu   Chengkun Qin   Chunyou Li , Baoxiang Hu   Shounan Yi , Xuefeng Xia , Haiqing Zhang, Xiujuan Zhang , Tingting Wang , Wenfei Pan , Chunxiao Yu , Qiangxiu Wang , Xiaoyan Lin   Laicheng Wang, Ling Gao Jiajun Zhao; Journal of Hepatology; 2015; Volume 62, Issue 5; pg 1171-1179.

The hypothalamus as a hub for putative SARS-CoV-2 brain infection; Sreekala Nampoothiri, Florent Sauve, Gaëtan Ternier, Daniela Fernandois, Caio Coelho, Monica Imbernon, Eleonora Deligia, Romain Perbet, Vincent Florent, Marc Baroncini, Florence Pasquier, François Trottein, Claude-Alain Maurage, Virginie Mattot, Paolo Giacobini, S. Rasika; BioRxIV; 2020.

Intersex and gender assignment; the third way? S F Ahmed, S Morrison, I A Hughes; Diseases in Childhood; 2004; volume 89; Issue 9.

Determination of the potency of a novel saw palmetto supercritical CO_2 extract (SPSE) for 5α-reductase isoform II inhibition using a cell-free in vitro test system; Pilar Pais, Agustí Villar, Santiago Rull; Research and Reports in Urology; 2016; 8: 41–49.

Growth and nutritional risk in children with developmental delay; C Malone, F Sharif , C Glennon-Slattery; Irish Journal of Medical Science; 2016;185(4):839-846.

Effect of early intervention in the developmental outcome of hypoxic ischemic encephalopathy infants: N. Meena1, Dr V.K. Mohandas kurup2, Dr. S. Ramesh3, Dr. R. Sathyamoorthy; IOSR Journal of Dental and Medical Sciences; 2014; Volume 13, Issue 3; PP 50-53.

Hypothalamic Menin regulates systemic aging and cognitive decline; Lige Leng, Ziqi Yuan, Xiao Su, Zhenlei Chen, Shangchen Yang, Meiqin Chen, Kai Zhuang, Hui Lin, Hao Sun, Huifang Li, Maoqiang Xue, Jun Xu, Jingqi Yan, Jie Zhang; PLoS Biology; 2023; 21(3): e3002033.

Physiology of BDNF: focus on hypothalamic function; Lucia Tapia-Arancibia, Florence Rage, Laurent Givalois, Sandor Arancibia; Frontiers in Neuroendocrinology; 2004; 25(2):77-107.

A GABAergic neural circuit in the ventromedial hypothalamus mediates chronic stress–induced bone loss; Fan Yang, Yunhui Liu, Shanping Chen, Zhongquan Dai, Dazhi Yang, Dashuang Gao, Jie Shao, Yuyao Wang, Ting Wang, Zhijian Zhang, Lu Zhang,1 William W. Lu, Yinghui Li, and Liping Wang; The Journal of Clinical Investigation; 2020.

Hypothalamic Menin regulates systemic aging and cognitive decline; Lige Leng, Ziqi Yuan, Xiao Su, Zhenlei Chen, Shangchen Yang, Meiqin Chen, Kai Zhuang, Hui Lin, Hao Sun, Huifang Li, Maoqiang Xue, Jun Xu, Jingqi Yan, Jie Zhang; PLOS Biology; 2023.

Morphofunctional Alterations of the Hypothalamus and Social Behavior in Autism Spectrum Disorders; Andrea Caria, * Luciana Ciringione, Simona de Falco; Brain Science; 2020; 10(7): 435.

Neuro-hormonal Regulation Is a Better Indicator of Human Cognitive Abilities Than Brain Anatomy: The Need for a New Paradigm; Arthur Saniotis, James P. Grantham, Jaliya Kumaratilake, Maciej Henneberg; Frontiers in Neuroanatomy; 2020; Volume 13.

Multi-level hypothalamic neuromodulation of self-regulation and cognition in preterm infants: Towards a control systems model; Sari Goldstein Ferber, Heidelise Als Gloria McAnulty Gil Klinger, Aron Weller; Comprehensive Psychoneuroendocrinology; 2022; Volume 9, 100109.

Remote effects of hypothalamic lesions in the prefrontal cortex of craniopharygioma patients; Jale Ozyurt, Anna Lorenzen, Ursel Gebhardt, Monika Warmuth-Metz, Hermann L Müller, Christiane M Thiel; Neurobiology of Learning and Memory; 2014;111:71-80.

Thyroid hormone and the developing hypothalamus; Anneke Alkemade; Front. Neuroanat. 2015; Volume 9.

The pathways from mother's love to baby's future; Aniko Korosi, Tallie Z. Baram; Frontier Behavioral Neuroscience; 2009.

Excessive Stress Disrupts the Architecture of a Child's Developing Brain; Takao Hensch et al; 2005.

Learning is a matter of history and relevance for lateral hypothalamus; Stan B Floresco; Nature Neuroscience; 2021; volume 24; 295-296.

Lateral Hypothalamus as a Motivation-Cognition Interface in the Control of Feeding Behavior; Gorica D. Petrovich; Frontiers of Systems Neuroscience; 2018; Volume 12.

The hypothalamus as a primary coordinator of memory updating; Denis Burdakov, Daria Peleg-Raibstein; Physiology & Behavior; 2020; Volume 223, 112988.

Peripheral Thyroid Hormone Conversion and Its Impact on TSH and Metabolic Activity; Holtorf, Kent; Journal of Restorative Medicine; 2014; Volume 3, Number 1, 30-52(23).

Physiology, Thyroid Hormone; Muhammad A. Shahid; Muhammad A. Ashraf; Sandeep Sharma. Stat Pearls; 2022.

Potential roles of mitochondrial cofactors in the adjuvant mitigation of proinflammatory acute infections, as in the case of sepsis and COVID-19 pneumonia; Giovanni Pagano, Carla Manfredi, Federico V. Pallardó, Alex Lyakhovich, Luca Tiano, Marco Trifuoggi; Inflammation Research. 2021; 70(2): 159–170.

The complex relationship between infertility and psychological distress (Review); Gabriela Simionescu, Bogdan Doroftei, Radu Maftei, Bianca-Elena Obreja, Emil Anton, Delia Grab, Ciprian Ilea, Carmen Anton; Experimental Therapeutic Medicine; 2021 Apr; 21(4): 306.

Is postural orthostatic tachycardia syndrome (POTS) a central nervous system disorder?; Svetlana Blitshteyn; Journal of Neurology; 2022; volume 269, pages 725–732.

A Review of Dietary (Phyto)Nutrients for Glutathione Support; Deanna M. Minich, Benjamin I. Brown; Nutrients; 2019; 11(9): 2073.

Drug abuse as a risk factor of multiple sclerosis: case-control analysis and a study of heterogeneity; L Brosseau, P Philippe, G Méthot, P Duquette, B Haraoui; Neuroepidemiology; 1993;12(1):6-14.

Childhood trauma in multiple sclerosis: a case-control study; Carsten Spitzer, Miriam Bouchain, Liza Y Winkler, Katja Wingenfeld, Stefan M Gold, Hans Joergen Grabe, Sven Barnow, Christian Otte, Christoph Heesen; Psychosomatic Medicine; 2012; 74(3):312-8.

Hypothalamic Dysfunction and Multiple Sclerosis: Implications for Fatigue and Weight Dysregulation; Kevin G. Burfeind, Vijayshree Yadav, and Daniel L. Marks; Current Neurology Neuroscience Reports; 2016; 16(11): 98.

Altered hypothalamic metabolism in early multiple sclerosis: MR spectroscopy study; Petra Hnilicová, Ema Kantorová, Hubert Poláček, Ján Lehotský, Dušan Dobrota, Egon Kurča; Journal of Neurological Sciences; 2019; 116458.

COVID-19 is associated with new symptoms of multiple sclerosis that are prevented by disease modifying therapies; Afagh Garjani, Rodden M Middleton, Rachael Hunter, Katherine A Tuite-Dalton, Alasdair Coles, Ruth Dobson, Martin Duddy, Stella Hughes, Owen R Pearson, David Rog, Emma C Tallantyre, Roshan das Nair, Richard Nicholas, Nikos Evangelou; Multiple Sclerosis Related Disorders; 2021; 52:102939.

Impact of Menopause in Patients with Multiple Sclerosis: Current Perspectives; Lorefice L, D'Alterio MN, Firinu D, Fenu G, Cocco; International Journal of Women's Health; 2023; Volume 15; 103-109.

Impact of Andropause on Multiple Sclerosis; Maria C. Ysrraelit, Jorge Correal; Frontiers in Neurology; 2021; 12: 766308.

Metals, autoimmunity and neuroendocrine; is there a connection? Geir Bjørklunda, Maryam Dadarb, Salvatore Chirumboloc,d, Jan Aasethe,f, Massimiliano Peanag; Environmental Research; 2020; 109541.

CDP-choline: Pharmacological and clinical review; J J Secades, G Frontera; Methods Find Experimental Clinical Pharmacology; 1995;17 Suppl B:1-54.

Leucine deprivation results in antidepressant effects via GCN2 in AgRP neurons; Feixiang Yuan et al; Life Metabolism; 2023.

Maternal pre-pregnancy body mass index is associated with newborn offspring hypothalamic mean diffusivity: A prospective dual-cohort study; Jerod M. Rasmussen, Jetro J. Tuulari, Saara Nolvi, Paul M. Thompson, Harri Merisaari, Maria Lavonius, Linnea Karlsson, Sonja Entringer, Pathik

D. Wadhwa, Hasse Karlsson & Claudia Buss; Boston Medical Center Medicine; 2023; 21, 57.

The role of prolactin in central nervous system inflammation; Edgar Ramos-Martinez, Ivan Ramos-Martínez, Gladys Molina-Salinas, Wendy A. Zepeda-Ruiz and Marco Cerbon; Reviews in the Neurosciences; 2021.

Adverse childhood experiences and chronic hypothalamic–pituitary–adrenal activity; Karen A. Kalmakis, Jerrold S. Meyer, Lisa Chiodo & Katherine Leung; Stress; 2015; 18:4, 446-450.

"Hypothalamic Microinflammation" Paradigm in Aging and Metabolic Diseases; Dongsheng Cai, Sinan Khor; Cell Metabolism; 2019; 30(1):19-35.

Viruses and Endocrine Diseases; Magloire Pandoua NekouaORCID, Cyril Debuysschere, Inès Vergez, Corentin Morvan, Chaldam Jespere Mbani, Famara Sane, Enagnon Kazali AlidjinouORCID and Didier Hober; Microorganisms 2023, 11(2), 361.

A microbiome-dependent gut–brain pathway regulates motivation for exercise; Lenka Dohnalová, Patrick Lundgren, Jamie R. E. Carty, Nitsan Goldstein, Sebastian L. Wenski, Pakjira Nanudorn, Sirinthra Thiengmag, Kuei-Pin Huang, Lev Litichevskiy, Hélène C. Descamps, Karthikeyani Chellappa, Ana Glassman, Susanne Kessler, Jihee Kim, Timothy O. Cox, Oxana Dmitrieva-Posocco, Andrea C. Wong, Erik L. Allman, Soumita Ghosh, Nitika Sharma, Kasturi Sengupta, Belinda Cornes, Nitai Dean, Gary A. Churchill, Christoph A.Thaiss; Nature; 2022.

Serotonin-estrogen interactions: What can we learn from pregnancy? Andrée-Anne Hudon Thibeault, J. Thomas Sanderson, Cathy Vaillancourt; Biochimie; 2019; Volume 161, 88-108.

Effect of progesterone on the expression of GABA(A) receptor subunits in the prefrontal cortex of rats: implications of sex differences and brain hemisphere; Susie Andrade, Bruno D Arbo, Bruna A M Batista, Alice M Neves, Gisele Branchini, Ilma S Brum, Helena M T Barros, Rosane Gomez, Maria Flavia M Ribeiro; Cell Biochemical Function; 2012; 30(8):696-700.

Central Regulation of PCOS: Abnormal Neuronal-Reproductive-Metabolic Circuits in PCOS Pathophysiology; Baoying Liao, Jie Qiao, Yanli Pang; Frontiers in Endocrinology (Lausanne); 2021; 12: 667422.

Dehydroepiandrosterone (DHEA) supplementation in diminished ovarian reserve;

Norbert Gleicher, David H Barad; Reproductive Biology and Endocrinology; 2011; 9: 67.

Dehydroepiandrosterone Sulfate (DHEAS) Levels in Polycystic Ovary Syndrome; Sikandar Hayat Khan, Syeda Arsheen Rizvi, Rahat Shahid, Robina Manzoor; Journal of College of Physicians Surgeons Pakistan; 2021; 31(3):253-257.

Anti-Müllerian Hormone and Inhibin-A, but not Inhibin-B or Insulin-Like Peptide-3, may be Used as Surrogates in the Diagnosis of Polycystic Ovary Syndrome in Adolescents: Preliminary Results; Aylin Yetim, Çağcıl Yetim, Firdevs Baş, Oğuz Bülent Erol, Gülnaz Çığ, Ahmet Uçar, Feyza Darendeliler; Journal of Clinical Research in Pediatric Endocrinology; 2016; 8(3):288-97.

Clinical Significance of Circulating C-Peptide in Diabetes Clinical significance of circulating C-peptide in diabetes mellitus and hypoglycemic disorders: A H Rubenstein, H Kuzuya, D L Horwitz; Archives of Internal Medicine;1977; 137(5):625-32.

Effect of umbilical cord essential and toxic elements, thyroid levels, and Vitamin D on childhood development; Jesse Cottrell, Chelsea Nelson, Catherine Waldron, Mackenzie Bergeron, Abigail Samson, Monica Valentovic; Biomedicine & Pharmacotherapy; 2023; Volume 158, 114085.

Emerging role of hypothalamus in the metabolic regulation in the offspring of maternal obesity; Jingyi Zhang, Sujuan Li, Xiaoping Luo; Cai Zhang; Frontiers in Nutrition; Sec. Nutrition and Metabolism; 2013; Volume 10.

Higher body mass index is linked to altered hypothalamic microstructure; K. Thomas, F. Beyer, G. Lewe, R. Zhang, S. Schindler, P. Schönknecht, M. Stumvoll, A. Villringer, A. V. Witte; Scientific Reports; 2019; volume 9, Article number: 17373.

Prolactin and autoimmunity; Luis J Jara, Gabriela Medina, Miguel A Saavedra, Olga Vera-Lastra, Carmen Navarro; Clinical Review Allergy Immunology; 2011; 40(1):50-9.

The role of prolactin in central nervous system inflammation; Edgar Ramos-Martinez, Ivan Ramos-Martínez, Gladys Molina-Salinas, Wendy A. Zepeda-Ruiz, Marco Cerbon; Reviews in the Neurosciences, 2020

The Interrelationship Between Serum Pituitary Hormones in Healthy Adults; Amit Akirov, MD; Endocrinology Advisor; 2020.

Late-onset hypogonadism: metabolic impact; M Grossmann, M Ng Tang Fui, A S Cheung; Andrology; 2020; 8(6):1519-1529.

Sex differences in the hypothalamic-pituitary-adrenal axis in patients with burning mouth syndrome; Lee YH, et al.; Oral Diseases; 2019.

Hypothalamus regulation of sleep and arousal; Ronald Szymusiak and Dennis McGinty; Molecular and Biophysical Mechanisms of Arousal, Alertness, and Attention; 2008; 1129(1): 275-286.

Hypothalamic inflammation: a double-edged sword to nutritional diseases; Dongsheng Cai and Tiewen Liu; Annuals New York Academy of Science; 2011; 1243: E1–39.

Hypothalamic-pituitary insufficiency following infectious diseases of the central nervous system; S Schaefer 1, N Boegershausen, S Meyer, D Ivan, K Schepelmann, and P H Kann; European Journal of Endocrinology; 2008; 158(1):3-9.

Adrenal insufficiency following traumatic brain injury in adults; David J Powner, and Cristina Boccalandro. Current Opinions in Critical Care; 2008; 14(2):163-6.

The Role of Circulating Amino Acids in the Hypothalamic Regulation of Liver Glucose Metabolism; Isabel Arrieta-Cruz and Roger Gutiérrez-Juárez; Advanced Nutrition; 2016; 7(4): 790S–797S.

Physiological adaptations to weight loss and factors favouring weight regain; F L Greenway; International Journal of Obesity (Lond); 2015; 39(8):1188–1196.

Menopause and the Human Hypothalamus: Evidence for the Role of Kisspeptin/Neurokinin B Neurons in the Regulation of Estrogen Negative Feedback; Naomi E. Rance; Peptide; 2009; 30(1): 111–122.

Hypothyroidism - new aspects of an old disease; I Kostoglou-Athanassiou and K Ntalles; Hippokratia; 2010; 14(2): 82–87.

The role of the hypothalamic-pituitary-adrenal axis in neuroendocrine responses to stress; Sean M. Smith, PhD; Dialogues Clinical Neuroscience; 2006; 8(4): 383–395.

Insulin and obesity transform hypothalamic-pituitary-adrenal axis stemness and function in a hyperactive state; Martin Werdermann, Ilona Berger, Laura D. Scriba, Alice Santambrogio, Pia Schlinkert, Heike Brendel, Henning Morawietz, Andreas Schedl, Mirko Peitzsch, Aileen J.F. King, Cynthia L. Andoniadou, Stefan R. Bornstein, and Charlotte Steenblock; Molecular Metabolism; 2021; 43: 101112.

The stimuli-specific role of vasopressin in the hypothalamus–pituitary–adrenal axis response to stress; Zelena, D., Domokos, Á., Jain, S. K., Jankord, R., & Filaretova, L.; Journal of Endocrinology, 2009; 202(2: 263-278.

Hair Loss and Hypothalamic–Pituitary–Adrenocortical Axis Activity; Novak MA, Hamel AF, Coleman K, Lutz CK, Worlein J, Menard M, Ryan A, Rosenberg K, Meyer JS; Journal of American Association of Laboratory Animal Science; 2014; 53(3):261-6.

The human hypothalamus in mood disorders: The HPA axis in the center; Ai-Min Bao, Dick F. Swaab, IBRO Reports; 2019; 6:45-53.

Gonadotropin levels can discern between hypothalamic hypogonadism, PCOS; Regina Schaffer; Healio; 2020.

A comprehensive review of the safety and efficacy of bioidentical hormones for the management of menopause and related health risks; Deborah Moskowitz; Alternative Medical Review; 2006; 11(3):208-23.

Hypothalamic integration of immune function and metabolism; Kim JH, Kim JH, Cho YE, Baek MC, Jung JY, Lee MG, Jang IS, Lee HW, Suk K.; Journal Proteome Research; 2014; 13(9):4047-61.

Changes in prolactin levels with the menopause; Schaefer S, Boegershausen N, Meyer S, Ivan D, Schepelmann K, Kann PH. European Journal of Endocrinology; 2008;158(1):3-9.

Berberine reduces insulin resistance induced by dexamethasone in theca cells in vitro; Zhao L, Li W, Han F, Hou L, Baillargeon JP, Kuang H, Wang Y, Wu X; Fertility and Sterility; 2011; 95(1):461-3.

Effects of berberine on glucose-lipid metabolism, inflammatory factors and insulin resistance in patients with metabolic syndrome; Cao C, Su M; Experimental and Therapeutic Medicine; 2019;17(4):3009-3014.

Hypothalamic oestrogen receptor alpha establishes a sexually dimorphic regulatory node of energy expenditure; J. Edward van Veen, Laura G. Kammel, Patricia C. Bunda, Michael Shum, Michelle S. Reid, Megan G. Massa, Douglas V. Arneson, Jae W. Park, Zhi Zhang, Alexia M. Joseph, Haley Hrncir, Marc Liesa, Arthur P. Arnold, Xia Yang, Stephanie M. Correa; Nature Metabolism; 2020; volume 2, pages 351–363

PART THREE

Mediterranean Diet on Sleep: A Health Alliance; Egeria Scoditti, Maria Rosaria Tumolo, Sergio Garbarino; Nutrients; 2022 Jul; 14(14): 2998.

Coffee consumption and health: umbrella review of meta-analyses of multiple health outcomes; Robin Poole, Oliver J Kennedy, Paul Roderick, Jonathan A Fallowfield, Peter C Hayes, Julie Parkes; British Medical Journal. 2018; 360: k194.

Health Risks and Benefits of Alcohol Consumption; Alcohol Research Health; 2000; 24(1): 5–11.

Contribution of Red Wine Consumption to Human Health Protection; Lukas Snopek, Jiri Mlcek, Lenka Sochorova, Mojmir Baron, Irena Hlavacova, Tunde Jurikova, Rene Kizek, Eva Sedlackova,Jiri Sochor; Molecules; 2018; 23(7): 1684.

Association between breakfast skipping and metabolic outcomes by sex, age, and work status stratification; Jun Heo, Won-Jun Choi, Seunghon Ham, Seong-Kyu Kang, Wanhyung Lee; Nutrition and Metabolism; 2021; Article number: 8.

Influences of Breakfast on Clock Gene Expression and Postprandial Glycemia in Healthy Individuals and Individuals with Diabetes: A Randomized Clinical Trial; Daniela Jakubowicz, Julio Wainstein, Zohar

Landau, Itamar Raz, Bo Ahren, Nava Chapnik, Tali Ganz, Miriam Menaged, Maayan Barnea, Yosefa Bar-Dayan, Oren Froy; Diabetes Care; 2017;40(11):1573-1579.

An Earlier First Meal Timing Associates with Weight Loss Effectiveness in A 12-Week Weight Loss Support Program; Mana Hatanaka, Yoichi Hatamoto, Eri Tajiri, Naoyuki Matsumoto, Shigeho Tanaka, Eiichi Yoshimura; Nutrients; 2022 Jan; 14(2): 249.

Dietary fat composition, total body fat and regional body fat distribution in two Caucasian populations of middle-aged and older adult women; Taulant Muka, Lauren C. Blekkenhorst, Joshua R. Lewis, Richar L. Prince, Nicole S. Erler, Albert Hofman, Oscar H. Franco, Fernando Rivadeneira, Jessica C. Kiefte; Clinical Nutrition; 2017, Volume 36, Issue 5, 1411-1419.

Three Minutes of All-Out Intermittent Exercise per Week Increases Skeletal Muscle Oxidative Capacity and Improves Cardiometabolic Health; Jenna B. Gillen, Michael E. Percival, Lauren E. Skelly, Brian J. Martin, Rachel B. Tan, Mark A. Tarnopolsky, Martin J. Gibala; PLOS One; 2014.

Cardiovascular Effects and Benefits of Exercise; Matthew A. Nystoriak, Aruni Bhatnagar; Frontiers in Cardiovascular Medicine; 2018; 5: 135.

Exercise modifies hypothalamic connectivity and brain functional networks in women after bariatric surgery: a randomized clinical trial; Carlos A. A. Merege-Filho, Saulo S. Gil, John P. Kirwan, Igor H. Murai, Wagner S. Dantas, Mariana P. Nucci, Bruno Pastorello, Alisson Padilha de Lima, Paulo R. Bazán, Rosa M. R. Pereira, Ana L. de Sá-Pinto, Fernanda R. Lima, Sonia M. D. Brucki, Roberto de Cleva, Marco A. Santo, Claudia da Costa Leite, Maria Concepción García Otaduy, Hamilton Roschel, Bruno Gualano; International Journal of Obesity; 2022; 47(3):1-10.

Hypothalamus-skeletal muscle crosstalk during exercise and its role in metabolism modulation; Kevin Ibeas, Laura Herrero, Paula Mera, Dolors Serra; Biochemical Pharmacology; 2021; Volume 190, 114640.

Sleeping with the hypothalamus: emerging therapeutic targets for sleep disorders; Emmanuel Mignot, Shahrad Taheri, Seiji Nishino; Nature Neuroscience; 2020; volume 5, 1071–1075.

The hypothalamic link between arousal and sleep homeostasis in mice: Tomoko Yamagata Martin C. Kahn, José Prius-Mengual, Vladyslav V. Vyazovskiy; Neuroscience; 2021.

Sleep disorders and the development of insulin resistance and obesity; Omar Mesarwi, MD, Jan Polak, Jonathan Jun, Vsevolod Y. Polotsky; Endocrinology and Metabolism Clinics of North America; 2013 Sep; 42(3): 617–634.

Neurological Evidence of a Mind-Body Connection: Mindfulness and Pain Control; Raymond St. Marie, M.D., Kellie S. Talebkhah, M.S.; Journal of Psychiatry, 2018.

 Mind and body: how the health of the body impacts on neuropsychiatry; Thibault Renoir, Kyoko Hasebe, and Laura Gray; Frontiers in Pharmacology. 2013; 4: 158.

Altered functional connectivity between hypothalamus and limbic system in fibromyalgia; Jian Kong, Yiting Huang, Jiao Liu, Siyi Yu, Cheng Ming, Helen Chen, Georgia Wilson, William F. Harvey, Wen Li & Chenchen Wang; Molecular Brain; 2021; volume 14, Article number: 17.

The Role of Circulating Amino Acids in the Hypothalamic Regulation of Liver Glucose Metabolism; Isabel Arrieta-Cruz, Roger Gutiérrez-Juárez, Nutrients. 2016; 7(4): 790S–797S.

Dietary Branched-Chain Amino Acids Regulate Food Intake Partly through Intestinal and Hypothalamic Amino Acid Receptors in Piglets; Min Tian, Jinghui Heng, Hanqing Song, Kui Shi, Xiaofeng Lin, Fang Chen, Wutai Guan, Shihai Zhang; Journal of Agricultural Food Chemistry; 2019; 67, 24, 6809–6818.

Amino acids and peptides of posterior pituitary and hypothalamus tissues; T. Winnick, R.E. Winnick, R. Acher, C. Fromageot; Biochimica et Biophysica Act; 1955: Volume 18, 488-494.

Amino Acid Levels in the Hypothalamus and Response to N-Methyl-D-Aspartate and/or Dizocilpine Administration during Sexual Maturation in Female Rats; Otero Losada M.E.·Carbone S.b·Szwarcfarb B.b·Moguilevsky J.A.; Neuroendocrinology 1993; 57:960–964.

Modulation of the hypothalamic-pituitary-adrenal (HPA) axis by plants and phytonutrients: a systematic review of human trials; Adrian L Lopresti, Stephen J Smith, Peter D Drummond; Nutritional Neuroscience; 2022; 25(8):1704-1730.

Therapeutic Effects of Phytochemicals and Medicinal Herbs on Depression; Gihyun Lee, Hyunsu Bae; Biomedical research international; 2017; 6596241.

Botanicals and Their Bioactive Phytochemicals for Women's Health; Birgit M. Dietz, Atieh Hajirahimkhan, Tareisha L. Dunlap, Judy L. Bolton; Pharmacological Reviews; 2016, 68 (4) 1026-1073.

n-3 Fatty Acids Induce Neurogenesis of Predominantly POMC-Expressing Cells in the Hypothalamus; Lucas F.R. Nascimento; Gabriela F.P. Souza; Joseane Morari; Guilherme O. Barbosa; Carina Solon; Rodrigo F. Moura; Sheila C. Victório; Letícia M. Ignácio-Souza; Daniela S. Razolli; Hernandes F. Carvalho; Lício A. Velloso; Diabetes; 2016;65(3):673-86.

Hypothalamic inflammation in obesity and metabolic disease; Alexander Jais, Jens C. Brüning; Journal of Clinical Investigations; 2017;127(1):24–32.

Training for Longevity: The Reverse J-Curve for Exercise; Evan L. O'Keefe, MD, Noel Torres-Acosta, MD, James H. O'Keefe, MD, Carl J Lavie, MD; Missouri Medicine. 2020; 117(4): 355–361.

Does Physical Activity Increase Life Expectancy? A Review of the Literature; C. D. Reimers, G. Knapp, A. K. Reimers; Aging Research; 2012; 243958.

An archival prospective study of mental health and longevity; Martin, L. R., Friedman, H. S., Tucker, J. S., Schwartz, J. E., Criqui, M. H., Wingard, D. L., & Tomlinson-Keasey, C.; 1995; Health Psychology; 14(5), 381–387.

Resources for Optimal Hypothalamus Health

Dear reader, you have just completed The Hypothalamus Handbook. I hope you found some wisdom within these pages and some practical tips to start healing the root of your health issues.

As promised, you can find additional resources at this link: https://genesis-gold.com/handbook

When you put your email in the link above, you will receive the following resources:

1. My Hypothalamus Questionnaire to fill out before going to your health care provider. This is all the information they will need from you to help come up with a diagnosis.

2. List of what to expect at your physical examination

3. List of blood work that I recommend to help diagnose hypothalamic dysfunction for both men and women.

4. My nutritional plans including my DMAR Nutritional Path to Wellness, my Liver Cleanse Diet, and my Insulin Resistance Diet

5. My CALM meditation

6. Information on Hormone Healing Circle, an online community that provides everything a hormonally challenged woman needs to heal

7. Discount Coupon for Genesis Gold, if you choose to utilize this as part of your hypothalamic healing regimen

Thank you for taking care of yourself physically, mentally, and spiritually. In healing your hypothalamus, the vibrations of healing will have a ripple effect. You'll notice that as you get better and more balanced, the people around you will begin to heal as well.

Love and Light,
Deborah Maragopoulos FNP
Intuitive Integrative Nurse Practitioner

About the Author

Deborah Maragopoulos FNP is an intuitive integrative family nurse practitioner who has spent over thirty years blending the Science of Medicine with the Art of Healing. Specializing in neuro-immune-endocrinology, Deborah focuses on optimizing the function of the hypothalamus - the maestro of the symphony of hormones. Deborah is a graduate of UCLA, the past president of the California Association of Nurse Practitioners, endocrine advisor for Genova Laboratories, founder of the charity Divine Daughters Unite and Genesis Health Products, and owner of Full Circle Family Health. Deborah is also author of the bestselling books Hormones in Harmony®, Menopause Action Plan, and Hypothalamus Handbook.

Printed in Poland
by Amazon Fulfillment
Poland Sp. z o.o., Wrocław

36324246R00150